The Doctor's Handbook, Part 1

The Doctor's Handbook, Part 1

MANAGING YOUR ROLE BEYOND CLINICAL MEDICINE

Fourth Edition

TONY WHITE

PhD FRCS MB BS AKC

Consultant Otolaryngologist (retired)

Foreword by

JOHN BLACK

President, Royal College of Surgeons

Radcliffe Publishing
Oxford • New York

Radcliffe Publishing Ltd
18 Marcham Road
Abingdon
Oxon OX14 1AA
United Kingdom

www.radcliffe-oxford.com
Electronic catalogue and worldwide online ordering facility.

First Edition 1999
Second Edition 2001
Third Edition 2006

British Library Cataloguing in Publication Data
A catalogue record for this book is available from the British Library.

ISBN-13: 978 184619 458 0

The paper used for the text pages of this book
is FSC certified. FSC (The Forest Stewardship
Council) is an international network to promote
responsible management of the world's forests.

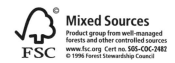

Mixed Sources
Product group from well-managed
forests and other controlled sources
www.fsc.org Cert no. SGS-COC-2482
© 1996 Forest Stewardship Council

Typeset by Pindar NZ, Auckland, New Zealand
Printed and bound by TJI Digital, Padstow, Cornwall, UK

Contents

Foreword

When you purchase a new computer there is never an instruction manual, other than brief instructions on the whereabouts of the on/off switch and how to clean the screen. This has led to bulging shelves in bookshops, packed with titles such as *Mac for Dummies: the manual you should have got with your computer but didn't*. At the onset of the two major steps in a medical career, namely into specialist training and consultant life, we could all do with an instruction manual, not about the clinical 'daytime job', difficult and challenging though it may be, but about the rest.

Part 1 is concerned with self-assessment and in the broadest terms improving professional communication at all levels. Much of this is taught in medical schools, but not brought together in an accessible way. Part 2 is a guide to the directorates, executive agencies, authorities, councils, departments, institutes and trusts that make up the modern NHS, together with insights into funding and a look into the future.

Every single thing in this book will turn up at some time in a specialist doctor's career, thankfully not all at once! Treat it as a *vade mecum* and guide to the complexities and frustrations of life as a medical specialist, which despite all remains an honourable and rewarding calling.

John Black
President
Royal College of Surgeons of England
May 2010

Preface

I often meet doctors who express the wish that they had received training earlier in their careers in a broader range of non-clinical aspects of their work. Others, who are committed to continuing professional development, seek learning material that will enable them to handle the wider issues they confront on a day-to-day basis, and for which initial medical education failed to prepare them. Many trainers can also find it difficult to access a single source that provides material for the non-clinical training of their juniors. This book, now in two parts, was written to address these and other needs revealed by research carried out by John Gatrell and me. Since publication I continue to be delighted with the positive feedback received from specialist registrars and other grades of doctors, including many consultants and surprisingly even NHS managers.

Before the first edition was published it was piloted extensively, working with doctors from many specialties. Many comments were received which helped to develop the first edition. John and I continued to receive positive feedback on the second and third editions and this has encouraged the publishers to go ahead with a fourth. With each new edition I have endeavoured to incorporate suggestions from readers. In this edition the chapters have been rearranged to allow new and existing material to be amalgamated where appropriate and make it easier to access information. It has been a difficult and rather subjective exercise which may not appeal to every reader.

Since the third edition, further changes in the structure, funding and governance of the NHS have continued, in addition to the changes that have occurred with the selection, training and appraisal of doctors. I have incorporated all these into this fourth edition, although inevitably there will be ongoing changes, for example, revalidation and Modernising Medical Careers (MMC), as they are carried through. At the time of writing many changes are imminent but not yet active; for example, the introduction of licensing and revalidation. This has obviously been a challenge in trying to be as up to date as possible between writing and publication.

To some extent I have tried to overcome this by referring the reader to the original source for current information. Indeed one of the striking changes in this edition compared to the original edition is the amount of information of value that is now available on various professional websites. Perhaps the most striking example is the information and guidance available from the General Medical Council website (www. gmc-uk.org) in almost all aspects of professional non-clinical work.

One criticism of the book has been a lack of some references but the number of direct references in the text is deliberate, as I want the text to be readable and informative. The book is not designed to be academic but rather to be a useful handbook.

Where no direct reference is quoted, you will find the sources of information in the related reading sections with each chapter.

I hope you will continue to find these books valuable in your current medical role and a means of support in your future professional development.

Tony White
May 2010

About the author

Tony White is a retired consultant otolaryngologist appointed in Bath, where he was clinical director for seven years. He has a PhD from Bath University with a thesis on 'The Role of Doctors in Management'.

Together with John Gatrell he undertook a three-year research project into the non-clinical development needs of doctors that resulted in publication of the NHS Training Directorate report, *Medical Student to Medical Director*, which also formed a basis for this book.

He has written several books on medical management and contributed to and edited several other textbooks as well as writing numerous papers. He has lectured widely and organised many workshops on doctors' management development issues. He was a member of a number of national advisory committees to develop doctors' non-clinical skills and acted as regular tutor on training courses in various regions.

Abbreviations

Latin abbreviations continue to be found in textbooks and learned journals. It is useful to know their meaning and indeed they may be used, albeit cautiously, in writing. I would suggest for clarity it is often better to write 'see above' and 'see below' rather than 'v. sup.' and 'v. inf'.

ad fin.	(*ad finem*) – near the end (of the page).
c./ca./cca.	(*circa*) – around, about, approximately, used of uncertain dates.
cap	(*capitulum*) – capital, capital letter or chapter.
cf.	(*confer*) – compare; used to suggest that another work might usefully be consulted in relation to the subject under discussion.
ead./eadem	see *id.*
e.g.	(*exempli gratia*) – for example, but sometimes used similarly to 'including' when not listing everything.
et al./*et al.*	(*et alii*) – and others. Used in multi-author references, although it is customary to include all the authors in the first citation and/or in the bibliography. It can also stand for *et alia* – and other things, or *et alibi* – and other places.
etc.	(et cetera) (include &c. and &/c.) – and the others, and other things, and the rest.
ff.	(*foliis*) – from pages used in citations to mean 'and on succeeding pages'.
i.a.	(*inter alia*) – among other things.
ibid./ib.	(ibidem) – in the same place; used in citations as 'in the same place' and relates to the immediately prior source.
id.	(*idem*) – the same (man). Used to avoid repeating the name of a male author (in citations, footnotes, bibliographies, etc.). If quoting a female author, use the corresponding feminine form *ead.* (*eadem*), the same (woman).
i.e.	(*id est*) – that is, or 'in other words'.
l.c./loc.cit.	(*loco citato*) – in the place already mentioned. Relates to sources before the immediately prior citation.
NB/n.b.	(*nota bene*) – note well.
op. cit.	(*opere citato*) – in the work already mentioned. Relates to sources before the immediately prior citation (loc. cit and op. cit. are more or less identical). In citations used in a similar way to 'ibid.', though 'ibid.' is usually followed by a page number.

p.m.a.	(*post mortem auctoris*) – after the author's death.
p.p./pp/*per pro.*	(*per procurationem*) – through the agency of.
PS/p.s.	(*post scriptum*) – written after.
q.v.	(*quod vide*) – which see; used to cross-refer to material that can be found elsewhere within a piece of writing. Note cf. refers to external material.
	For more than one term or phrase, the plural is *quae videre* (qq.v.).
seq./seqq.	(*sequentia*) – the following.
sc./scil.	(scilicet = *scire licet*) – that is to say or namely.
sic	– indicates that text is literally transcribed from the original. Often written in parentheses following a misspelled word to indicate that the error is the original writer's mistake.
s.v.	(*sub voce*) – under the word (specified). Used with alphabetically arranged reference works.
v.	(*vide*) – see, look up.
v. inf.	(*vide infra*) – see below.
viz	(videlicet) – that is to say, namely. As distinct from i.e. and e.g., viz. is used to indicate a detailed description of something stated before, and when it precedes a list of group members, it implies near completeness.
v.s. v.sup.	(*vide supra*) – see above.
vs.	(versus) – against.

Acknowledgements

I remain especially grateful to Dr Hugh Platt, whose vision initiated and inspired the original work.

My thanks are also due to those readers who took the trouble to contact us with suggestions for this fourth edition.

I wish to thank those who provided wisdom and guidance over all the editions including medical royal colleges, postgraduate deaneries, medical defence organisations, health authorities and hospital and primary care trusts. I freely acknowledge that some ideas may have come from seeds sown during discussions with these people. I apologise if any reference is not attributed or is incorrectly acknowledged; any such errors are mine alone.

Particular thanks in this edition are due to Liz Jones for her help in finding, writing and checking material and for stepping in at a very late stage, working into the small hours, to write new material for clinical governance and quality. Jenny Barker, Managing Director, Wiltshire PCT, for advice and checking of facts. Tim Albert, writer and trainer, for general advice on writing skills. Gillian Nineham of Radcliffe Publishing, the midwife who coped with a rather difficult birth of this fourth edition.

Due to other commitments John Gatrell has not been able to act as co-author for this edition. In his place I have received help and guidance from colleagues working in the various subjects. But it is appropriate to express thanks for the efforts he has given to earlier editions and for his provision of useful new material such as that on Meyers-Briggs personality types, emotional intelligence and the writings of Frederick Herzberg.

Not least, I am grateful to my wife Anne not only for her efforts in checking and researching new material, but whose continued support, tolerance and encouragement has made the whole fourth edition possible.

Tony White

Introduction

These handbooks have three main aims:

○ to support the development of a range of mainly non-clinical skills related to professional development

○ to provide a basis for making the most of a number of learning opportunities that occur during training

○ to serve as a source of useful information to doctors in the NHS.

Sometimes it is difficult to ask for advice about non-clinical aspects of our work – it is often assumed that we should acquire this awareness through a kind of osmosis, picking it up along the way. The books try to provide answers to questions that you feel you ought to know, but perhaps do not like to ask. The books also provide assistance with the development of new skills and capabilities that we know are relevant to professional careers. It is intended to be a useful resource to help you with a particular problem and an opportunity to work through larger sections in order to learn more about specific aspects of your work.

Some kinds of learning can be achieved through reading textbooks, some through one-to-one instruction and others are better undertaken in group training sessions. All require opportunity and an element of underpinning knowledge with a commitment to learn. These handbooks are designed to cover the knowledge element that is the basis for developing professional skill and judgement. It should fit in with your work and be relevant to everyday needs. It supplements other training such as short courses which become available from time to time.

The books emerged from an extensive study of the non-clinical learning needs of doctors at all stages in their careers and has been further informed by a series of development programmes for doctors. The General Medical Council's 'Good Medical Practice Guidelines' remind us that a high level of clinical competence is only one aspect of professional medical practice. Personal insight, effective team working, good leadership, teaching others and skill in dealing with patients need to be supported by clear understanding of the complex structures and systems in the modern NHS.

Following the introduction of MMC, standardised multi-source feedback techniques have been introduced to improve the assessment of interpersonal skills exhibited by doctors in training. This is just one example of the increased breadth of assessment that modern medical trainees must be able to accommodate. Their world has increased in complexity through technological advances on the one hand and political intervention on the other. As future consultants they may be expected to play a much greater role in the organisations in which they work, yet have less power and influence than most of their predecessors. I have tried to cover a wide range of needs in these books. I hope you find it useful and enjoy the experience of using them as a learning resource.

Needs and experience change over time and it would be helpful if you let me know things that need to be included, things that could be omitted and things that need changing or moving from one section to another. This process of continuous development and review will ensure that it stays relevant for future readers.

Learning objectives

Key learning objectives of these handbooks are listed below. You might find it helpful to start by familiarising yourself with their contents as a whole. If you believe you are already competent in an area, study the action points in that section. This should help you to decide if you need to do more. You may feel that some sections are irrelevant at this stage in your career. Put them to one side, but make a note to return to them later. These books will also act as a reference document into which you can dip as the need arises.

On completion of the books you should be better able to do the following.

o Identify your preferred learning style and make better use of learning opportunities.
o Organise your time so that you can cope with work and enjoy available leisure time.
o Delegate tasks to others in a way that helps to develop them and permits you to make better use of your own abilities.
o Make effective presentations to small and large groups.
o Work efficiently in a team.
o Lead others in the achievement of team goals.
o Understand and deal with conflict.
o Deal with stress in yourself and others.
o Contribute usefully and effectively to meetings.
o Instruct and train others in skills and knowledge aspects of clinical tasks.
o Appraise and assess in the context of training and revalidation.
o Present clear and concise formal reports and other written communications.
o Undertake research and prepare articles for publication.
o Present yourself successfully in the selection process.
o Deal with patients and close family members when breaking bad news.
o Request a post mortem.
o Appear at a coroner's inquest and as a witness in court.
o Support and advise colleagues and help them to develop.
o Identify the key aspects of quality service delivery.
o Recognise trust and related national systems for risk management.
o Differentiate between audit and research and apply audit principles to a range of settings.
o Reflect on your personal values in the context of your career and work as a doctor.
o Understand something of the current structure and funding of the NHS.
o Have a clearer idea of the way healthcare is changing and developing.

Exploring your approach to working and learning

The aim of this chapter is to enable you to increase your self-awareness. It will help you to reflect on your approach to your work and the impact you have on colleagues and patients, and to explore your preferred learning style.

What type of doctor are you?

A doctor usually works in a number of trusts, firms or jobs as they proceed through training. This gives them an opportunity to learn about the differing sets of values and attitudes that tend to be a feature of a particular organisation. As they become employees of each, they may consider how well their own values relate with those of their colleagues in each place. Older generations of doctors sometimes regard doctors in training as being less able and committed than they themselves were at a similar stage in their careers and are inclined to believe that changing attitudes to work will have a negative effect on patients. Without perfect recall we (and they) are unable to prove or disprove this perspective. A high level of self-insight is undoubtedly an important asset for those developing their professional competence and standing.

The following questionnaire enables you to reflect on the values you bring to the organisation in which you work. It may also help you to understand more about other doctors with whom you work. You might find it interesting to carry out a quick self-diagnostic questionnaire to assess your own values in the context of your work as a doctor. It may also be beneficial for you to repeat it after you are appointed as a consultant and consider any changes that have occurred. The questionnaire is introduced here to help you to get some feedback about your approach to your role as a doctor in comparison to other approaches that you might take. It also gives some insight into how doctors might be perceived in their hospital and how others with whom they work might judge their impact.

The questionnaire is derived from *Doctors and Dilemmas* by Mascie-Taylor, Pedler and Winkless (1996), and is used with their permission.

Read each statement and place a tick in the box corresponding to the one option out of the four presented that most applies to you.

Question	A	B	C	D
In the development of my work people would describe me as . . .				
. . . striving on behalf of the whole.			☐	
. . . uninvolved.	☐			
. . . a good corporate citizen.			☐	
. . . a fighter for my own service.				☐
As a consultant I . . .				
. . . should not be seen to have to lead very often.	☐			
. . . should lead from the front (and not expect to be questioned a great deal).		☐		
. . . lead by creating a vision for the hospital/department and motivating others.			☐	
. . . have an important role within my team.				☐
My colleagues would tend to say of me that . . .				
. . . I am the sort of person who is likely to initiate and deal well with change.			☐	
. . . I can be relied upon to look after my patients, and play my part in the team.				☐
. . . I am perhaps a bit of a character and occasionally selfish and pushy.		☐		
. . . they tend not to talk or know much about me.	☐			
As a consultant it will be important for me to . . .				
. . . look after my patients, and be supportive of the hospital.				☐
. . . look after my patients and develop my service and specialty.		☐		
. . . look after my patients and avoid wasting time doing other things.	☐			
. . . look after my patients and contribute ideas for the development of the hospital.			☐	

Question	A	B	C	D
I believe it is important for research to be carried out in the hospital . . .				
. . . so long as it does not interfere with patient care or divert one away from outside interests.	☐			
. . . so that doctors can treat patients more effectively.				☐
. . . so as to improve patient services which the hospital offers and to enhance its reputation.			☐	
. . . so that the reputation of individual doctors and their specialty is enhanced.		☐		
As a future consultant I . . .				
. . . should be a leader of my team where appropriate.				☐
. . . should not be concerned to any great extent with leading others.	☐			
. . . should become a leader of my specialty.		☐		
. . . should be a leader in the hospital.			☐	
In my non-clinical working relationships with others in the hospital I . . .				
. . . single-mindedly pursue the self-interest of my specialty.		☐		
. . . do not have many relationships with others.	☐			
. . . attempt to work with others to the best of my ability.				☐
. . . attempt to show others that there is a brighter future.			☐	
In dealing with patients I . . .				
. . . resist any restriction which a shortage of resources might bring about.		☐		
. . . just get on with dealing with an individual patient.	☐			
. . . make sure the hospital as a whole responds as well as possible to the needs of patients.			☐	
. . . recognise that there are issues beyond the individual patient.				☐
When I attend a management course, my interest would be in . . .				
. . . how to make a team work more effectively, contributing to others and the hospital.				☐
. . . leadership and strategic management.			☐	
. . . understanding the system so that I can get what I want.		☐		
. . . very little of what was on offer.	☐			

Question

	A	B	C	D
I believe the curriculum for medical students should comprehensively cover . . .				
. . . more medical topics and less of the 'social sciences'.			☐	
. . . methods of effective team working.				☐
. . . strategic management of the NHS.			☐	
. . . managing the doctor–patient relationship.	☐			
In terms of my leadership style I . . .				
. . . like to join with people and participate.				☐
. . . tell people what they need to know.		☐		
. . . consult, then seek to influence.			☐	
. . . have never really thought about it much.	☐			
Modern management practices in the NHS . . .				
. . . must be resisted at all times by the medical profession.		☐		
. . . have a useful place.				☐
. . . are only vaguely understood by me.	☐			
. . . offer the key to the future.			☐	
My views of managers in the NHS is that they . . .				
. . . are partners in the management of a complex organisation.			☐	
. . . are irrelevant to my practice.	☐			
. . . are an unnecessary imposition.		☐		
. . . have a part to play and contribution to make.				☐
In my view, service commissioners . . .				
. . . should find the funds to enable my specialty to expand.		☐		
. . . should be seen as partners in the strategic development of our hospital.			☐	
. . . should ensure balance in developments even if it affects my specialty negatively.				☐
. . . seem very remote and beyond my sphere of influence.	☐			
As a consultant, financial considerations should . . .				
. . . be none of my concern.	☐			
. . . be of importance.			☐	
. . . be vigorously resisted if they get in the way of my service.		☐		
. . . have a part to play.				☐

Question	A	B	C	D
As a consultant if I was invited by the chief executive to a meeting to discuss significant cost reductions which might affect my clinical practice I would . . .				
. . . either not attend the meeting or attend and say nothing.	❑			
. . . attend, recognising that to resolve the issue requires a team-working approach.				❑
. . . attend in order to make positive suggestions for taking the hospital forward.			❑	
. . . attend in order to minimise the effect on my specialty.		❑		
In discussions with my colleagues about the resource implications of practice I . . .				
. . . accept that resource limitations are part of the ethical debate.				❑
. . . take the view that practice guidelines should not be influenced by resource implications.		❑		
. . . persuade other clinicians of the need to seek solutions to such dilemmas.			❑	
. . . tend not to venture a view.	❑			
As a consultant I would like my professional work to be recognised for . . .				
. . . strongly influencing the direction of the hospital.			❑	
. . . providing a good service.				❑
. . . solely my clinical work.	❑			
. . . being influential in the profession.		❑		
I feel that primary care as a service commissioner . . .				
. . . has shifted power from hospital doctors in an inappropriate way.		❑		
. . . emphasises the need for consultants in directorates to work together.				❑
. . . is irrelevant to my practice.	❑			
. . . has created hospitals which require strategic leadership.			❑	
If it were suggested that the hospital in which I was working should merge with another, in the interests of patient care I would . . .				
. . . only support the merger if I thought that my own specialty would benefit.		❑		
. . . contact my opposite numbers in the other unit to help in forging an effective new alliance.			❑	

Question	A	B	C	D
. . . support the merger in the light of the common good.				☐
. . . recognise that I would have little influence on the outcome.	☐			

My view of attending conferences is that they . . .

	A	B	C	D
. . . can be useful for networking effectively with other influential doctors and managers.			☐	
. . . are essential for meeting and influencing other important doctors in my specialty.		☐		
. . . are not normally part of my life or practice.	☐			
. . . are something I do in order to keep up to date.				☐

The leadership of clinical services . . .

	A	B	C	D
. . . rests with the doctor as far as my patients are concerned.	☐			
. . . is a medical role with some important managerial implications.			☐	
. . . should be shared on the basis of professional expertise.				☐
. . . is the doctor's right.		☐		

A primary care-led NHS . . .

	A	B	C	D
. . . makes me work with colleagues to meet GPs' needs.				☐
. . . is doomed to failure since it removes power from those who really understand.		☐		
. . . is a piece of jargon which I don't really understand.	☐			
. . . represents a strategic opportunity for the hospital which should be embraced.			☐	

Consultant job plans are . . .

	A	B	C	D
. . . helpful for consultants to work together.				☐
. . . an unnecessary imposition by management on consultant practice.		☐		
. . . unnecessary given the straightforward nature of consultant work.	☐			
. . . a useful tool in ensuring that objectives of a hospital are met.			☐	

What I admire most in my colleagues is . . .

	A	B	C	D
. . . their ability to lead.			☐	
. . . the way they are not distracted from their daily clinical work.	☐			
. . . their ambition for themselves and their specialty.		☐		
. . . their being prepared to contribute to the team effort.				☐

Question	*A*	*B*	*C*	*D*

I would like to think that my obituary in the *BMJ* will say . . .

. . . I was first and last an outstanding clinician. ☐ *(A)*

. . . I was primarily an outstanding medical manager. ☐ *(C)*

. . . I was primarily outstanding in my specialty. ☐ *(B)*

. . . I was primarily outstanding in working in a team for the good of the patient. ☐ *(D)*

Analysis of your questionnaire responses

The ticks for your answers fall under columns headed A, B, C, or D. Add up the total scores for the whole questionnaire for each column and enter into the boxes.

☐　　　☐　　　☐　　　☐
A　　　B　　　C　　　D

Your highest score suggests one of four possible positions that doctors take with regard to the resolution of common dilemmas that arise in fulfilling their role. Doctors manage at various levels, their personal practice, in teams and groups, departments and units and other places. Full details of the use of a Repertory Grid approach to this analysis can be found in Mascie-Taylor, Pedler and Winkless (1996) who produced four ideal type descriptions or 'identikits' (*see* Figure 1.1).

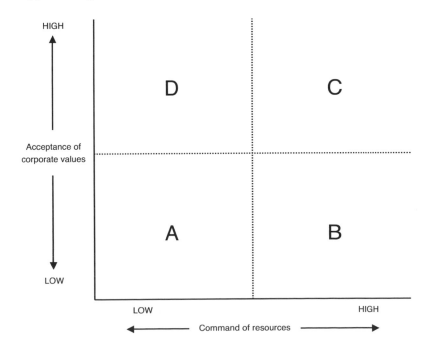

FIGURE 1.1 Types in relation to resources and corporate values

Caricatures emerge with clarity, but type A turns out to include a variety of subtypes. A cautionary note: people vary in the way they respond to questionnaires by tending to score lowly, highly or opting for the middle option. Also, each question is given equal weight, so the salience of questions for you may not be fairly represented. You need to remember these points, particularly if you are making comparisons with other people.

What type are you?
Type 'D': the TEAM PLAYER – 'the good corporate citizen'
Focus:
- primarily on the team but with awareness and interest in the whole organisation
- team leader advising rather than leading the organisation.

Abilities and skills:
- takes leadership at team level and is prepared to accept it at corporate level
- plays by rules within corporate goals, a building block of the organisation
- participative, co-operative, loyal, supportive, shares responsibilities, a team worker
- good interpersonal skills, good communicator
- economical with resources
- personable, well respected.

Beliefs and values:
- service orientation
- recognises the added value and complementary skills of management
- democratic process, participation, consultation
- loyalty to medicine and medical values together with valuing the whole organisation.

Implications:
- the backbone of the organisation
- dedicated clinicians – the 'sort you'd like to take your mother to'
- interested in playing their part in the whole
- lack confidence or have insufficient skills to be Type C leaders
- less inclined to take risks than Type C leaders
- prefer to avoid tough decisions
- may choose the quiet life
- may pursue outside interests
- may focus on the medical role
- less likely than Type C leaders to take on formal management roles
- careful with resources
- may be self-sacrificing in meeting demands of others.

Type 'C': the LEADER – 'who strives on behalf of the whole'
Focus:
- commitment to the organisation
- wide view, broad vision, strategic thinking.

Abilities and skills:
○ agent of change, politically astute
○ high interpersonal skills, influential, good communicator, good listener, assertive and can be tough
○ manages resources on behalf of the whole
○ develops people and teams
○ manages conflict, is constructive and supportive, tolerant of ambiguity and dilemmas.

Beliefs and values:
○ quality service and value for money requires doctors and managers to work together
○ capability in the whole system is what counts
○ pluralistic, different sources of loyalty are legitimate, conflict is inevitable
○ endemic and needs to be managed
○ people (including self) are developing beings and can learn.

Implications:
○ the managers may regard you as too good to be true and lacking a 'shadow side'
○ although Type Cs are often highly committed and very able leaders, Type Bs and perhaps Type As may see them as having 'gone over to the other side', or as having failed to make it in medicine and are now seeking an alternative career
○ some Type Cs may be Type Bs in temporary disguise, playing the corporate game in order to secure advantage; others may indeed be more interested in personal career advancement than with the rather altruistic 'good of the whole' – a strong motivation may be the desire to learn and explore new possibilities, not just of career but of person
○ Type Cs are widely liked and respected for their leadership qualities, especially by Type Ds.

Type 'B': the INDEPENDENT – 'who fights for their own patch'
Focus:
○ me and my specialty
○ me and my profession.

Abilities and skills:
○ confidence, dominance, determined, may be aggressive
○ political skills, well connected, knows the 'right people'
○ entrepreneurial, energetic and hard working
○ uses conflict
○ has good ideas, sometimes functional and sometimes dysfunctional for organisation.

Beliefs and values:
○ self-belief and self-worth
○ individuality, individual excellence is what counts

o specialty is all-important
o doctors don't need managing but need administration
o rules are to be broken, or 'my rules'.

Implications:
o little in the way of corporate loyalty or values
o uninterested in corporate management
o see managers (at best) as means of acquiring resources for their patch
o often lack sensitivity to others and may appear aloof, overbearing or arrogant
o arouse strong feelings of admiration, or fear or dislike
o express themselves well in advancing their own work or specialty, but are poor at team work, chairing meetings or achieving agreement
o can be extrovert, convivial and amusing
o ability to command resources in the hospital or via external funding while lacking an awareness and concern for the whole makes them often the most difficult people to manage.

Type 'A': the CONTRACT CLINICIAN – 'uninvolved'
Focus:
o one-to-one patient care and clinical management with no particular interest, awareness or involvement beyond this.

This is a collection of subtypes. Classified as low on both corporate values and command of resources, this type has few abilities, skills, beliefs or values which are relevant from a leadership or managerial perspective.
o **A1: the new starter** – The junior doctor on the way to Type B, C or D. May be naive, idealistic, dedicated and with little awareness of how the hospital or health services work and with little energy or attention to spare for learning the role.
o **A2: the disengager** – Winding down and preparing to separate from the organisation through retirement, tiredness or ill-health.
o **A3: the contract worker** – The doctor working 'nine to five' who doesn't want to get involved in anything outside one-to-one patient care. May have domestic responsibilities or consuming interests outside work. Does a job for the hospital within the strict limits of the contract.
o **A4: the isolate** – The loner who may be good, bad or indifferent, but is essentially unrecognised in terms of contribution. May work in remote location or specialty or be isolated for some other reason.

Implications:
o Type As have least impact because they do little to the organisation as a whole beyond their immediate task. This is not a commentary on them as people or as doctors; they may be effective or ineffective at that task. They may be learners or about to retire, they may have a limited contractual relationship with the organisation, or have a deep moral involvement in patient healthcare. They share a certain

isolation from the run of events and may be candidates for further personal and professional development.

Action

Note your type now and consider what this means for you, your colleagues, the hospital and your future in healthcare. You may find it instructive to repeat this questionnaire at the end of your first year as a consultant and consider how you have changed and why.

Learning and problem solving – what is your preferred style?

This section seeks to give insight into some concepts behind teaching and learning. An understanding of the thinking behind training methods being used today will help you to get the most from your learning opportunities. I think it would be helpful to introduce you to the work of Kolb, Osland and Rubin (2000).

Career development and the maintenance of professional competence demand that doctors maintain learning habits throughout their working lives. Most of us associate learning with the process we followed at school and university, when tutors provided us with knowledge, often through lectures to large groups of students, and concepts which we dutifully wrote down and memorised and fed back in the essays and project work and examination questions completed as a means of assessing our learning. End-of-term, end-of-year and final examinations helped to confirm the view that demonstrating learning involved satisfying others – our assessors – that we had grasped the necessary *concepts*.

Necessary for what, though? 'Life', as you will already have realised, in the form of daily work with patients, requires a different approach, where problem solving requires us to gain *experience*, quite different from the unreal world of classroom learning. The concept of learning as we came to know it during school and university often seems less relevant now.

The concept of problem solving also suggests an active rather than passive process. In other words the responsibility for problem solving rests with you, in contrast to teaching, where the teacher is responsible (for the learning). The problem solver must experiment, take risks and gain experience, in order to address the problem.

This separation of *educational* learning and *work* learning sometimes leads to difficulties for doctors in the transition from medical school to work-based training. Our preferred approaches to learning are usually based on early, school-based experience, which do not always match later learning needs. This section will try to:

o illustrate this concept
o identify your preferred learning style
o show how various learning styles are relevant to different situations
o provide a model for learning which will help you to take full advantage of learning opportunities as they arise

○ help you to understand why you find some kinds of learning more acceptable than others.

The inventory below is for describing how you learn – the way you find out about and deal with ideas and situations in your life. Different people learn best in different ways. The different ways of learning described in the survey are all equally good. The aim is to describe *how* you learn, not to evaluate your learning ability. You might find it hard to choose the descriptions that best characterise your learning style. Keep in mind that there are no right or wrong answers – all the choices are equally acceptable.

Learning-style inventory
Source: Kolb, Osland and Rubin (2000), used with permission (*see* related reading list, p. 25).

Instructions
There are nine sets of four descriptions listed in this inventory. Mark the words in each set that are most like you, second most like you, third most like you, and least like you. Put a four (4) next to the description that is *most* like you, a three (3) next to the description that is *second* most like you, a two (2) next to the description that is *third* most like you, and a one (1) next to the description that is *least* like you (4 = *most* like you; 1 = *least* like you). Be sure to assign a different rank number to each of the four words in each set; *use whole numbers only.*

Example
4 happy   **3** fast   **1** angry   **2** careful

(Some people find it easiest to decide first which word best describes them (**4** happy) and then decide the word that is least like them (**1** angry). Then you can give a 3 to that word in the remaining pair that is most like you (**3** fast) and a 2 to the word that is left over (**2** careful).

1 _ discriminating	_ tentative	_ involved	_ practical
2 _ receptive	_ relevant	_ analytical	_ impartial
3 _ feeling	_ watching	_ thinking	_ doing
4 _ accepting	_ risk taker	_ evaluative	_ aware
5 _ intuitive	_ productive	_ logical	_ questioning
6 _ abstract	_ observing	_ concrete	_ active
7 _ present-oriented	_ reflecting	_ future-oriented	_ pragmatic
8 _ experience	_ observation	_ conceptualisation	_ experimentation
9 _ intense	_ reserved	_ rational	_ responsible

Scoring instructions
The four columns of words correspond to the four learning-style scales: **CE** (concrete experience), **RO** (reflective observation), **AC** (abstract conceptualisation) and **AE** (active experimentation). To compute your scale scores, write your rank numbers in the

boxes below only for the designated items. For example, in the third column (**AC**), you would fill in the rank numbers you have assigned to items 2, 3, 4, 5, 8 and 9. Compute your scale scores by adding the rank numbers for each set of boxes.

score items: 2 3 4 5 7 8	score items: 1 3 6 7 8 9	score items: 2 3 4 5 8 9	score items: 1 3 6 7 8 9
----------------	----------------	----------------	----------------
Total: **CE** = _____	Total: **RO** = _____	Total: **AC** = _____	Total: **AE** = _____

When the characteristics of learning and problem solving are combined, it is possible to come to a closer understanding of how people use their experience to develop concepts, rules and principles that guide their behaviour in new situations. The process can be conceived as a four-stage cycle, as shown in Figure 1.2.

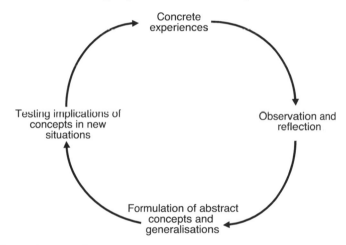

FIGURE 1.2 Four-stage cycle

○ *Concrete experience* is any experience which has an impact, either physical or emotional, on the person. It is normally as a result of interaction with others that we feel such an impact. This is followed by
○ *Observation and reflection* on the experience, taking time to make sense of the context and the experience itself. This should then lead to the formation of
○ *Abstract concepts and generalisations*, or explanations which help us to explain the nature and reasons for our reactions to the experience. We may then test out our reasoning by
○ *Active experimentation*, or trying out new behaviours and approaches in the fourth stage. This leads on to further experience, and so on.

The model shows learning as a continuously recurring cycle. All learning is relearning, and all education is re-education. It may also be assumed that learning is shaped by personal needs and goals, which affect the ways in which we interpret experience.

Thus, learning is likely to be erratic and inefficient when personal objectives are not clear.

Interpreting your scores on the learning-style inventory

The learning-style inventory (LSI) is a simple self-description test based on experiential learning theory. It is designed to measure your strengths and weaknesses as a learner in the four stages of the learning process. Effective learners use four different learning modes: concrete experience (CE), reflective observation (RO) abstract conceptualisation (AC) and active experimentation (AE).

One way to understand the meaning of your scores on the LSI is to compare them with the scores of others. The target diagram in Figure 1.3 gives the norms on the four basic scales (CE, RO, AC, AE) for 1933 (American) adults ranging from 18 to 60 years of age. About two-thirds of the group are men and the group as a whole is well educated (two-thirds have university degrees or higher). A wide range of occupations and educational backgrounds are represented. They include teachers, engineers, managers, doctors and lawyers.

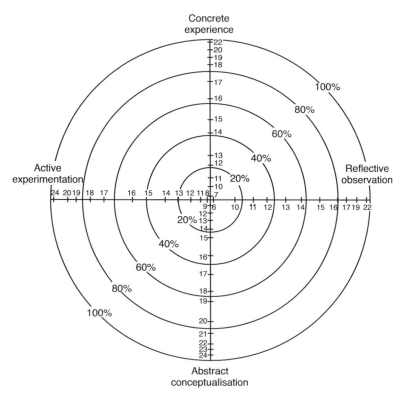

FIGURE 1.3 Learning-style profile norms (© David A Kolb (1976))

The raw scores for each of the four basic scales are marked on the crossed lines of the target. By marking your raw scores on the four scales and connecting them with straight lines you can create a graphic representation of your learning-style profile. The concentric circles on the target represent percentile scores for the normative group.

It should be emphasised that the LSI does not accurately define your learning style. It is an indication of how you see yourself as a learner. Your scores indicate which learning modes you emphasise in general. They may change from time to time and situation to situation.

The inventory is designed to give you some indication of which learning modes you tend to emphasise. No mode is better or worse than any other. Even a totally balanced profile is not necessarily best. The key to effective learning is being competent in each mode when it is appropriate.

Orientation towards *concrete experience* suggests being involved in experiences and dealing with immediate human situations in a personal way. It emphasises *feeling* as opposed to *thinking*, and concern with the uniqueness and complexity of present reality as opposed to theories and models, an intuitive, artistic approach as opposed to a systematic, scientific approach to problems. People with concrete experience orientation enjoy and are good at relating to others. They can be good intuitive decision makers, and function well in unstructured situations. They value highly relationships with people and being involved in real situations, and they keep an open-minded approach to life.

An orientation towards *reflective observation* emphasises comprehending the meaning of ideas and situations by carefully observing and impartially describing them. It emphasises understanding as opposed to practical application. Such people enjoy thinking about the *meaning* of situations and ideas, and are good at discovering their implications. They often look at things from different perspectives and appreciate different points of view. They value patience, impartiality and considered, thoughtful judgement, and tend to rely on their own thoughts and feelings to form opinions.

Orientation towards *abstract conceptualisation* focuses on using logic, ideas and concepts. It emphasises thinking as opposed to feeling, and is concerned with building general theories rather than intuitive understanding. Such a person enjoys and is good at systematic planning, manipulation of abstract symbols, and quantitative analysis. They value precision, the rigour and discipline of analysing ideas, and the aesthetic quality of a neat conceptual system.

An orientation towards *active experimentation* focuses on actively influencing people and changing situations. It emphasises practical applications as opposed to reflective understanding, and a pragmatic concern with what works as opposed to what is absolute truth. Such people enjoy and are good at getting things accomplished. They are willing to take some risk to achieve their objectives. They also value having an impact and influence on the environment around them, and like to see results.

Action

Greater insight into your preferred learning style should provide you with a basis for exploiting learning opportunities. If possible, discuss your profile with that of colleagues. Compare and contrast them, and consider if it helps to explain your previous performance in learning situations and different subject areas.

Identifying your learning-style type

It is useful to describe your learning style by a single data point that combines your scores on the four basic modes. This is accomplished by using the two combination scores, **AC** minus **CE** and **AE** minus **RO**. These scales indicate the degree to which you emphasise *abstract* over *concrete* and *action* over *reflection*, respectively.

The grid shown in Figure 1.4 has the raw scores for these two scales on the crossed lines (**AC–CE** on the vertical and **AE–RO** on the horizontal) and percentile scores based on the normative group on the sides. By marking your raw scores on the two lines and plotting their point of interception, you can find which of the four learning-style quadrants you fall into.

These four quadrants, labelled *accommodator*, *diverger*, *converger* and *assimilator*, represent the four dominant learning styles. If your **AC–CE** score were −4 and your **AE–RO** score were +8, you would fall strongly in the accommodator quadrant. An **AC–CE** score of +4 and an **AE–RO** score of +3 would put you only slightly in the converger quadrant. The closer your data point is to the point where the lines cross, the more balanced your learning style.

If your data point is close to any of the four corners, this indicates that you rely heavily on one particular learning style.

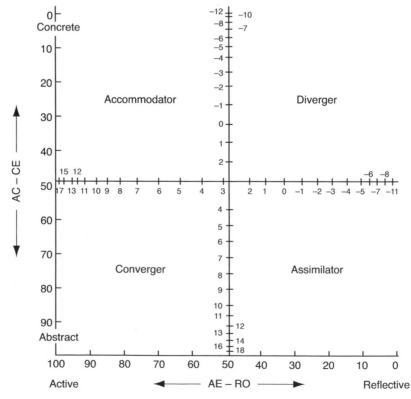

FIGURE 1.4 Learning style type grid (© David A Kolb (1976))

The following is a description of the characteristics of the four basic learning styles based both on research and clinical observation of these patterns of LSI scores.

o The **convergent** learning style relies primarily on the dominant learning abilities of abstract conceptualisation and active experimentation. The greatest strength of this approach lies in problem solving, decision making and the practical application of ideas. This learning style is called 'converger' because a person with this style seems to do best in such situations as conventional intelligence tests where there is a single correct answer or solution to a question or problem. In this learning style, knowledge is organised in such a way that, through hypothetical-deductive reasoning, it can be focused on specific problems. Liam Hudson's research on individuals with this style of learning shows that convergent persons are controlled in their expression of emotion. They prefer dealing with technical tasks and problems rather than with social and interpersonal issues. Convergers have often specialised in the physical sciences. This learning style is characteristic of many engineers and technical specialists.

o The **divergent** learning style has the opposite strengths of the convergent style, emphasising concrete experience and reflective observation. The greatest strength of this orientation lies in imaginative ability and awareness of meaning and values. The primary adaptive ability in this style is to view concrete situations from many perspectives and to organise many relationships into a meaningful 'Gestalt'. The emphasis in this orientation is on adaptation by observation rather than by action. This style is called 'diverger' because a person of this type performs better in situations that call for generation of alternative ideas and implications such as a 'brainstorming' idea session. Persons oriented towards divergence are interested in people, and tend to be imaginative and feeling oriented. Divergers have broad cultural interests and tend to specialise in the arts. This style is characteristic of individuals from humanities and liberal arts backgrounds. Counsellors, organisation development specialists and personnel managers tend to be characterised by this learning style.

o In **assimilation**, the dominant learning abilities are abstract conceptualisation and reflective observation. The greatest strength of this orientation lies in inductive reasoning, in the ability to create theoretical models and in assimilating disparate observations into an integrated explanation. As in convergence, this orientation is less focused on people and more concerned with ideas and abstract concepts. Ideas, however, are judged less in this orientation by their practical value. Here it is more important that the theory be logically sound and precise. This learning style is more characteristic of individuals in the basic sciences and mathematics rather than the applied sciences. In organisations, persons with this learning style are found most often in the research and planning departments.

o The **accommodative** learning style has the opposite strengths of assimilation, emphasising concrete experience and active experimentation. The greatest strength of this orientation lies in doing things, in carrying out plans and tasks, and in getting involved in new experiences. The adaptive emphasis of this orientation is on opportunity seeking, risk taking and action. This style is called 'accommodation' because it is best suited for those situations in which one must adapt oneself to changing immediate circumstances. In situations where the theory or plans do not fit the facts, those with an accommodative style will most likely discard the plan or theory. (With the opposite learning style, assimilation, one would be more likely to disregard or re-examine the facts.) People with an accommodative orientation tend to solve problems in an intuitive trial-and-error manner, relying on other people for information rather than on their own analytical ability. Individuals with accommodative learning styles are at ease with people, but are sometimes seen as impatient and 'pushy'. This person's educational background is often in technical or practical fields such as business. In organisations, people with this learning style are found in 'action-oriented' jobs, often in marketing or sales.

Self-awareness

Insight into yourself and the way others see you can be a difficult thing to acquire. This is made more difficult for people in training to achieve high professional status, because boasting about strengths is not usually seen as acceptable and admitting weaknesses can feel quite threatening to career development.

The 'Johari window', named after the first names of its inventors, Joseph Luft and Harry Ingham, is one of the most useful models describing the process of human interaction. It is often used, as here, to demonstrate an approach to developing insight into oneself through interaction with close colleagues. A four-paned 'window', as illustrated in Figure 1.5, divides personal awareness into four different types, as represented by its four quadrants: open arena, hidden, blind spot and unknown potential. The lines dividing the four panes can move as an interaction progresses.

The **open arena quadrant** represents things that I know about myself and that others know about me. The knowledge that the window represents can include not only factual information but also my feelings, motives, behaviours and perhaps some of my wishes. When I first meet a new person, the size of the opening of this first quadrant is not very large, since there has been little time to exchange information. As the process of getting to know one another continues, the dividers move down or to the right, placing more information into the open window, as described below.

The **blind spot quadrant** represents things that others know about me, but of which I am unaware. Others may know, for example, that I have said something that upset a colleague because he has complained to them, but if no one tells me, I remain unaware of the offence I have caused. This information is in my blind quadrant because others can see it, but I cannot. If someone now tells me that I have upset my colleague, the window shade moves to the right, enlarging the open quadrant's area. Now, I may also have blind spots with respect to many other much more complex things. For example, perhaps in conversation, my eye contact seems to be lacking. Colleagues may say nothing, in order to avoid embarrassing me by implying that I am being insincere. The problem is: how can I get this information out in the open since it may be affecting the level of trust that is developing between my colleagues and me? How can I learn more about myself? I may notice a slight discomfort showing in the person I am talking to, and perhaps this may lead to a question. It is difficult for me to identify the problem unless someone else makes me aware of it.

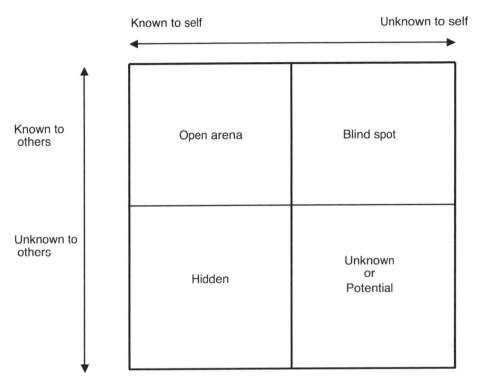

FIGURE 1.5 The Johari window

The **hidden quadrant** represents things that I know about myself that others do not know. So, for example, if I have not told my colleagues that I enjoy golf, this information is in my hidden quadrant. As soon as I share my love of the sport, I am effectively pulling the window shade down, moving the information in my hidden quadrant and enlarging the open quadrant's area. Again, there are perhaps vast amounts of information, virtually my whole life's story, that have yet to be revealed to my colleagues. As we get to know and trust each other, I will then feel more comfortable disclosing more intimate details about myself. This process is called: 'self-disclosure'.

The **unknown potential quadrant** represents things that neither I nor others know about me. This may include experiences that affect my behaviour and that lie deep in my subconscious and which I may never come to know. Or, I may have the potential to achieve excellence in playing a musical instrument, but because I have never been offered, or have availed myself, of the opportunity, I, with others, remain unaware of this. Sometimes, a novel situation can trigger new awareness and personal growth. I may find myself having to cope with a new, unexpected challenge that I discover I enjoy and can meet with relative ease. The process of moving previously unknown information into the open quadrant, thus enlarging its area, can often be likened to achieving self-fulfilment.

Giving and receiving feedback is something that requires a high level of skill and confidence that takes time to develop. The Johari window demonstrates that seeking feedback and disclosing information about ourselves in order to elicit feedback from others has the effect of enlarging the open quadrant. Typically, as I share something about myself (moving information from my hidden quadrant into the open), and if the other party is interested in getting to know me, they will reciprocate, by similarly disclosing information in their hidden quadrant. Thus, an interaction between two parties can be modelled dynamically as two active Johari windows. It helps to choose someone you feel you can trust and whose response will give you some insight into yourself.

As your level of confidence develops, you may actively invite others to comment on your blind spots. You may already seek feedback from students on the quality of a particular lecture, with the desire of improving the presentation. The next stage is to invite comment on your ability to deal with more complex aspects of your role. Self-disclosure – giving the other person something about yourself that helps to build mutual confidence and trust – is an excellent way to start.

The practical aspects of feedback and effective listening are discussed more fully in Chapter 3, 'Effective interpersonal communication skills'.

Myers-Briggs Personality Type Indicator

Psychometric tests are used increasingly in the NHS for training and development purposes. Understanding our preferred ways of behaving and mapping these on to others' preferences can be helpful in that it increases our self-awareness and the impact we may have on others. It also helps us to understand why others behave in the way they do.

One of the best known and most widely used is the Myers-Briggs Type Indicator (MBTI). You might have encountered it in a team or leadership development programme in the latter stages of your training. Based on a theory of personality types first developed by Carl Jung in the early 1900s, it works on the principle that, although everyone is unique, there are patterns in people's behaviour that are predictable and consistent. Katherine Briggs and her daughter Isabel Myers developed this theory over a lifetime and, after 30 years of refinement, produced a self-completed questionnaire that helps people identify their own preferences.

A guiding principle of the MBTI is that there are no right or wrong types, all are relevant and valuable and only the individual can decide his or her own type. It has been used extensively to improve the way people work together in organisations. It has great potential for helping doctors on a personal level and is used for such things as personal and career development, improving team working and colleague relationships and understanding stress.

The attraction of the MBTI is that it provides a very simple framework to describe four important ways in which people differ, but it also allows room for great depth and complexity.

The MBTI reports people's preferred ways of behaving on four scales, each consisting of two opposite poles. These four scales are as follows.

1   Where we prefer to focus our attention – either in the outside world (extroversion), or in our heads (introversion).
2   The way we prefer to take in and process information – either literally and logically (sensing), or generally and in broad patterns (intuition).
3   The kinds of information we prefer to prioritise in decision making – either logical and objective (thinking), or value-based and people-oriented (feeling).
4   Our preferred style of living and working – either scheduled or organised (judging), or spontaneous and flexible (perceiving).

The easiest way to explain what is meant by 'preference' is to sign your name with your usual hand and then do the same thing with the other hand. Writing with your usual hand feels easy and natural, while the other feels awkward and difficult. The same applies to behaviour preferences – you can do it the other way, but it feels less natural and you would probably need to practise for a while before you could get the same result. You can imagine how difficult and tiring it would be if you had to use your non-preferred hand all day. Jung believed that preferences are inborn, but that the extent to which we develop them is affected by our environment and experience of life.

It is important to recognise that the meanings attributed to these words are not necessarily those we would use in everyday language today. For instance, 'judging' does not mean being judgemental in the sense of making negative assessments of people or things. Rather, it refers to a preference for making decisions.

Scale 1
Extroversion (E)
People who tend towards extroversion are energised by active involvement in events, and they like to be immersed in a wide range of activities. They are most excited when they are around people and they often have an energising effect on those around them. Extroverts like to move into action and to make things happen.

Introversion (I)
People who prefer introversion are energised when they are involved with the ideas, images, memories and reactions that are a part of their inner world. Introverts often prefer solitary activities or spending time with one or two others with whom they feel an affinity and they often have a calming effect on those around them.

Scale 2
Sensing (S)
People who have a preference for sensing are likely to be seen as more grounded in everyday physical reality. They tend to be concerned with what is actual, present, current and real. As they exercise their preference for sensing, they approach situations with an eye to the facts. Thus, they often develop a good memory for detail, become accurate in working with data and remember facts or aspects of events that did not even seem relevant at the time they occurred. For sensing types, experience speaks louder than words or theory.

Intuition (N)

People who have a preference for intuition are immersed in their impressions of the meanings or patterns in their experiences. They would rather gain understanding through insight than through hands-on experience. Intuitive types tend to be concerned with what is possible and new and they have an orientation to the future. They are often interested in the abstract and in theory and may enjoy activities where they can use symbols or be creative.

Scale 3

Thinking (T)

People who have a preference for thinking judgement are concerned with determining the objective truth in a situation. More impersonal in approach, thinking types believe they can make the best decisions by removing personal concerns that may lead to biased analyses and decision making. The thinking function is concerned with logical consistency and analysis of cause and effect. As they use and develop their thinking function, thinking types might appear analytical, cool and tough-minded.

Feeling (F)

People who have a preference for feeling judgement are concerned with whether decisions and actions are worthwhile. They believe they can make the best decisions by weighing what people care about and the points of view of persons involved in a situation. Feeling types are concerned with personal values and find it easier to put themselves in the place of those who may be affected by their decisions – which are usually based on what is best for the people involved.

Scale 4

Judging (J)

People who have a preference for judging use their preferred judging function (whether it is thinking or feeling) in their outer life. They will appear to prefer a planned or orderly way of life; for example, to have things settled and organised, feel more comfortable when decisions are made and like to bring life under control to the degree that it is possible.

Perceiving (P)

People who have a preference for perceiving use their preferred perceiving function (whether it is sensing or intuition) in their outer life. What this often looks like is that they prefer a more flexible and spontaneous way of life and like to stay open to new experiences. They enjoy rushing to meet deadlines but avoid fixed plans whenever possible. They like to keep their options open to allow for the unexpected.

Personality types

Our preference in each pair determines our personality type based on these preferences. Thus, for example, an ISTJ type is likely to be practical, serious and earn success through thoroughness and dependability. They are logical in decision making and prefer order and structure in their lives. They have a preference for written communication and are unlikely to be the first to contribute to meetings, preferring to consider carefully before committing.

An ENFP type is likely to be enthusiastic, spontaneous and flexible, ready to proceed based on the patterns they see rather than the detail. Face-to-face discussion is their preferred means of communication and they depend on their ability to improvise and their verbal fluency.

Reliability and validity

The Myers-Briggs Type Indicator questionnaire was tested exhaustively for its reliability and validity during the 30 years of development. Measures of internal consistency, together with test-retest reliability coefficients, have shown reliabilities in excess of 80. High correlations were found between specific parameters of the MBTI, such as introversion and extroversion, and other psychometric instruments, but more interestingly the MBTI was found to predict reliably both self-assessed and observed behaviour for all eight of the Myers-Briggs preferences and was also found to be predictive of other aspects of psychology, such as conformity versus independence, focus on achievement, happy families, preference for variety and challenge, achievement and so on. These tests have been repeated for the UK version of the MBTI.

In the UK, a licensed practitioner who has been selected and trained by the authorised supplier of the relevant materials should normally undertake Myers-Briggs profiling. If an opportunity arises to learn about your own Myers-Briggs profile, you are advised to take it up as the insight gained from a better understanding of the impact we have on others and why others affect us as they do can make us much more effective in our work.

Related reading

Allen J, Brock SA. *Health Care Communication Using Personality Type*. London: Routledge; 2000.

Berens LV. *Understanding Yourself and Others: an introduction to temperament*. California: Telos; 2000.

Briggs-Myers I, revised by Kirby LK, Myers KD. *Introduction to Type*. Oxford: OPP; 2000.

Evans C. *Time Management for Dummies*. Chichester: Wiley; 2008.

Houghton A. Understanding personality type: introducing personality type. *BMJ Career Focus*. 2004; **328**: 177–8.

Kolb DA, Osland JS, Rubin IM. *Organizational Behaviour: an experiential approach*. 6th ed. Englewood Cliffs, NJ: Prentice-Hall; 2000.

Maitland I. *Managing Your Time*. London: Chartered Institute of Personnel and Development; 1999.

Mascie-Taylor HM, Pedler MJ, Winkless AJ. *Doctors and Dilemmas: a study of 'ideal types' of doctor/managers and an evaluation of how these could support values of clarification for doctors in the health service*. Bristol: NHSTD; 1996.

Teaching, training, appraisal, assessment and revalidation

This chapter will guide you through various aspects of teaching, learning and training. It also covers various forms of appraisal and assessment, licensing and revalidation, mentoring, counselling and career guidance and, finally, poorly performing colleagues.

This chapter, probably more than any other, has required the most radical review for this edition. A great deal has changed in the training, appraisal and assessment of doctors for those in training and for consultants. There is also the added task of revalidation and relicensing.

Teaching and training

Continuing medical education and professional development is fundamental to career progress. This follows the principles required for safe and effective practice in line with the codes of *Good Medical Practice* (GMC 2006). There is often confusion about the meaning of the terms 'teaching' and 'training'. Definitions for the purposes of this handbook are outlined below.

Is there a difference between teaching and training, and if so what are they? Teaching as defined by various dictionaries has many definitions, including causing to know, enabling, tell or show how, to guide the studies of, to impart the knowledge of. Training similarly defined implies bringing a person to a desired standard by instruction and practice, or preparing for a test of skill.

Note that training focuses on skill as the definitions imply a narrower focus than teaching and possibly a shorter timeframe. We might associate training with the notion of procedures that we repeat until we develop the skills we are trying to acquire. The definitions for teaching imply deeper knowledge and a longer timeframe. We talk about lifelong learning, but not about lifelong training.

Competence and confidence

There is evidence to suggest that confidence levels (but not skill levels) grow with experience alone. An interesting paper (Marteau *et al.* 1990), published in the BMJ and available to download online even if you are not a member, demonstrated that experience by itself is insufficient to develop competence. And another more recent paper assessing basic life support (BLS) confidence as assessed against competence (Castle *et al.* 2007) of doctors in training, qualified nurses and healthcare assistants (HCAs) suggested similar findings.

Learning

We tend to think of learning as a formal process, although much real learning is informal. It occurs on a day-to-day basis without our being particularly aware of it. This process was discussed in Chapter 1. Much time is wasted when the needs and preferences of the teacher rather than the needs of the learner decides the method used. A better basis for choice would be that based on learning domains, of the material to be learned.

Learning domains

The nature of the task to be learned can vary in content and complexity, which can influence the approach to teaching. The following categorisation of learning situations represents a simple way of helping to decide which approach to teaching is likely to be most helpful to the learner.

There are three major learning domains: cognitive, affective and psychomotor. The education of doctors and the practice of medicine, as with other professionals in medicine, engage all three.

o **Cognitive** (knowing or understanding)

The acquisition of knowledge, concepts and intellectual skills and abilities. Developed through reading, studying, and question-and-answer and discussion sessions.

o **Psychomotor** (skills)

▸ *Practical skills* – requiring co-ordinated activity and precise manipulative procedures, they involve practice in order to acquire competence (from suturing to endoscopy and surgical procedures). Usually achieved through instruction and guided practice. This is what doctors often think of when referring to training. Instruction may be as short as three or four minutes. Periods of skills training of more than about 15 minutes can be difficult. Doctors generally want to be involved and to start using newly learned skills.

▸ *Interpersonal skills* – these are more complex skills often employed when dealing with people (colleagues or patients, individuals or groups), allaying patients' concerns, displaying empathy, trust and respect for colleagues and upholding high ethical standards. Interpersonal skills are of considerable importance in teamwork, including handling conflict, influencing, counselling and information gathering (history taking). Such skills are more difficult to impart. Demonstration, role playing and feedback using video can be helpful. Doctors often find it difficult to admit, often to themselves, that they need help in dealing with others. Most believe they are good at communicating. As is so often the case, insight is the first stage in learning. You can read more about communication skills in Chapter 3.

o **Affective** (feelings, attitudes, emotions, mindsets and values)
Based on complex sets of values and beliefs, desirable attitudes for personal and professional development (allaying patient concerns, displaying empathy, trust and respect with colleagues, upholding high ethical standards in practice). Acquired throughout life, they are dependent on a wide range of influences, family, friends and colleagues, particularly 'role models', also partly on the influence of those who impress us during our formative learning stages. Seniors almost certainly influenced your attitudes to many aspects of your work, perhaps even your choice of career. In turn you will help to shape the attitudes of more junior colleagues. Indeed, you might even help shape the attitudes of some of your senior colleagues. Teaching and training require developed skills. Every time you help others to learn, try to get feedback on your own performance.

Teaching

Teaching for this book is taken to mean pre-arranged sessions in which one person makes a formal presentation of learning material to a group. They usually only attempt the one-way transfer of information and not skills. It may be in the form of a teacher-led discussion or a formal lecture. There's an old academic joke that describes the latter as an activity during which the notes of the lecturer are transferred to the notebooks of the students without passing through the minds of either!

The aim of teaching is the hope and expectation that at least some of the audience will leave with an improved understanding or level of knowledge. Your responsibility as a teacher is to select, arrange and deliver to meet that expectation. So it is good to start by defining the needs of the audience rather than what you want to tell them.

You then need to find and use ways of making your teaching interesting and relevant. Presentational skills can be developed (attending a training course or by practising and getting feedback from reliable members of your audiences). Chapter 3 on interpersonal communication will give you further guidance on presentation techniques.

Sensible use of audiovisual aids is important. PowerPoint can guide a lecturer like a drunk going from lamppost to lamppost and some teachers feel that students take it as a cue to tune out. It can also make a lecture scripted and linear and there is just a 'forced march' through the material. So careful planning is important; it is also important to remember the value of audience participation as this can help create effective teaching sessions.

Training

Training is different to teaching as it is a two-way process of instruction that tends to focus on skills rather than knowledge. Thus it has a narrower focus and usually a shorter timeframe, perhaps repeating a procedure where the skill is acquired. Training is best performed on a one-to-one basis. Just as with teaching, it requires planning.

o Resources should be available to complete the session. This involves the room, equipment, perhaps patients and the necessary paperwork in addition to allowing yourself sufficient time.
o Check that the current level of capability of trainees is appropriate for their needs. By discussing their needs, motivation to learn will be increased.
o Have learning goals or objectives for the session. These should be agreed with the trainee and stated in measurable terms.
o Method of instruction. This is dealt with in more detail below.
o Evaluation. How will you measure success? Preferably before the instruction starts and with agreement of trainee.
o Record of completion and achievement of the learning goals for logbook.
o Support and follow-up. It is important that learners are given time to master their new skills and not left on their own without support and guidance being available during the early practice stages.

Method of (skills) training

Surgical training in which skills training is particularly relevant is changing: a hundred years of tradition is challenged by increasing legal and ethical concerns for patient safety, restrictions on working hours (European Working Time Directive – EWTD) and the cost of theatre time in a target-driven environment.

Surgical simulation and skills training now offer an opportunity to teach and practise advanced skills outside the theatre setting before attempting them on living patients. Simulation training can be as simple as using real instruments and video equipment to manipulate simulated 'tissue' in a box. But more advanced, virtual reality simulators are now becoming available and ready for use. However, the need still exists for a common method for skills training. One that has stood the test of time is the **'four-step' procedure** and most methods are a variation on this theme. It is based on breaking down large, complex tasks into smaller elements. The trainee can then be shown and can practise each stage separately before attempting the whole task as one.

The four steps are as follows, with questions only after each run-through.

1 The trainer performs the task with the trainee observing.
2 The trainer performs the task again while talking through each stage. There are three steps within this one.
   a Tell them what you are going to do.
   b Tell them while you are doing it.
   c Take time to deal with further questions after you have done it.
3 The trainee talks through the task while the trainer performs it. This gives the trainer an opportunity to check understanding.
4 The trainee performs the task and talks it through at the same time. Consolidation of learning begins at this stage. There is also the opportunity to stop the trainee from making a mistake before it occurs. This is critically important in some situations (e.g. in an operating theatre, where the trainee would explain each step and get clearance from the trainer before proceeding).

Giving effective feedback is a key part of the training process. It is not always done well and the following guidelines for giving feedback will help in most situations.
○ Be positive, encouraging and supportive.
○ Be specific and deal clearly with particular incidents and examples of behaviour. Avoid vague comments.
○ Suspend judgement. It is unhelpful to pronounce judgement but better to say how you see the situation and let the trainee make their own evaluation.
○ Make it actionable. It is not helpful to give someone feedback about something that they cannot change. Useful feedback can lead to a change in behaviour.
○ To be most effective, feedback needs to be given as soon after the event as practical so it is fresh in the receiver's mind.
○ Praise may be given in front of others.
○ Negative feedback is generally best left until you can deal with it on a one-to-one basis.

Assume that trainees will continue to need your support for some time after the training session as it would be an unusual trainee who got everything right first time. This may at first involve direct supervision until they can be left alone to perform the task. Always explain how you or some other suitable person can be contacted until the trainee feels entirely competent.

Appraisal

The first problem we have with appraisal is that the terminology is confused and confusing. For example, it is often used for similar processes by different colleges. If asked for a short definition of appraisal, the briefest found is: a process to provide feedback on doctors' performance, chart their continuing professional development (CPD), and identify their developmental needs. Sometimes feedback on appraisal of performance is referred to as formative assessment. In order to avoid confusion I have tried to use all the terms rather than confine myself to one strict definition. So appraisal, sometimes known as formative assessment, has the aim of providing developmental and educational feedback to you by your appraiser.

Educational appraisal is a developmental formative process that is trainee-focused. The training for individual trainees should be optimised, taking into account available resources and the needs of other trainees. Educational appraisal is defined in the NHS 'Gold Guide' (2007 edition) as a positive process to provide feedback on the trainee's performance, charting their continuing progress and identifying their developmental needs (after The New Doctor transitional edition, 2005). Workplace-based (NHS) appraisal is the process whereby trainees are appraised by their educational supervisors on behalf of their employers, using the assessments and other information which have been gathered in the workplace. Training opportunities must meet the training standards as set by the Postgraduate Medical Education and Training Board (PMETB) and should be viewed as a continuous process. As a minimum, the educational element of appraisal should take place at the beginning, middle and end of each section of training, normally marked by the Annual Review of Competence Progression process. However, appraisal may be needed more frequently; for example, after an assessment outcome that has identified inadequate progress.

Appraisal ought to be regarded as developmental rather than judgemental and therefore it is normally confidential. It should allow a trainee to openly discuss any concerns about their performance and future career plans. A well-conducted trainee appraisal meeting should provide the opportunity for the trainee to gain important new insights in discussion with a senior colleague whose opinion is important to them. The appraiser is helping a trainee to reflect, acquire and develop an understanding of new concepts. The appraisal allows the trainee to go out and test their learning in their own way (under supervision) and acquire further new experiences to reflect on.

Appraisal is based around the General Medical Council's document *Good Medical Practice* (GMC 2006), which describes the principles of good medical practice, and the standards of competence, care and conduct expected of doctors in all aspects of their professional work. These are:

o good clinical care
o maintaining good medical practice
o teaching and training
o relationships with patients
o working with colleagues
o probity
o health.

The first heading, good clinical care, is specialty-specific and medical royal colleges and specialty groups have provided guidance. For the majority of trainees, the information provided will be their College Logbook and assessment documents. Trainee appraisal is part of an educational process, although it has an element of performance review. It is essential that it is open, objective, subject to appeal and properly designed to inform decisions about career progress.

The other headings of GMP are common to all doctors and, again, medical royal colleges and specialty groups have provided guidance. For consultants, appraisal should be maintained as a formative (educational) process (BMA 2008), providing positive information for revalidation, such as participation in CPD. It should be conducted as a developmental, rather than a punitive, process.

About the same time and just after the NHS Clinical Governance Support Team (CGST) had co-ordinated the training of appraisers in primary care, the idea for a website to support appraisal for doctors arose. The website is now defunct but based on the idea in 2008 NHS CGST set up the Revalidation Support Team (RST), also a Department of Health-funded body, to support the implementation of revalidation. Its aims were as follows.

o Provide leadership for the design and delivery of new appraisal arrangements in England.
o Work with stakeholders on the piloting, evaluation and implementation of appraisal.

○ Ensure professions, employers and commissioners are informed and involved in design and rollout of the new arrangements.
○ Work closely with the Devolved Administrations to ensure consistency of approach where possible and appropriate.

The Revalidation Support Team tries to engage with other major stakeholders; for example, the GMC, the Academy of Medical Royal Colleges (AMRC), the individual colleges, strategic health authorities, and many others including the British Association of Medical Managers (BAMM). With pilots to test revised appraisal processes, it tries to develop and inspire the confidence of the profession in the process.

Then there are organisations that have been formed to help in the appraisal process, such as UK Appraisal and Revalidation Support (UKARS), an independent organisation set up to support revalidation for healthcare professionals in the UK. Its members are healthcare professionals who have been working with the NHS Clinical Governance Support Team and the Career Grade Doctor Appraisal Forum (CGDAF), both of which have published a series of documents about appraisal on the website at www.appraisalsupport.nhs.uk. Separate from the DoH, GMC, the AMRC and its constituent colleges and faculties, UKARS says it works closely with them and is funded by some of them. Initial work has focused on the appraisal of doctors, but the scope of activity is being increased to include supporting all aspects of the revalidation of doctors (*see* p. 51). They also work with other health professions as they introduce regulatory processes.

Appraisal for general practitioners was introduced in England in 2002, in Northern Ireland and Scotland in 2003 and in Wales in 2004. In all cases it was constructed primarily as a formative and developmental process. In 2007 the DoH published a series of documents and guidance on Appraisal for GPs and these can be viewed at www.dh.gov.uk/en/Managingyourorganisation/Humanresourcesandtraining/EducationTrainingandDevelopment/Appraisals/DH_4052082. Although some of the documents are dated as far back as 2002, one entitled 'Appraisals – Questions and Answers – GPs' is quite useful and was updated in 2007.

There is also a website for consultants at www.dh.gov.uk/en/Managingyourorganisation/Humanresourcesandtraining/EducationTrainingandDevelopment/Appraisals/DH_4051692. It will provide you with some useful guides updated in 2007.

Because there are differing appraisal systems for different groups of doctors, and it is not possible to reproduce everything here, you are advised to visit a comprehensive Department of Health website at www.dh.gov.uk/en/Managingyourorganisation/Humanresourcesandtraining/EducationTrainingandDevelopment/Appraisals/index.htm. This has links to appraisals as well as links to appraisal questions and answers and sharing best practice, as follows:
○ in general
○ for GPs
○ NHS clinical consultants
○ academic clinical consultants
○ consultants in public health medicine

- non-consultant career-grade doctors
- doctors in training in the NHS
- Whole Practice Appraisal – appraisal for doctors with a private practice.

Continuing professional development

The GMC make it clear that doctors have a responsibility to keep up to date. It will be one of the criteria for NHS appraisals and revalidation with the GMC who have a statutory role promoting high standards and co-ordinating all aspects of medical education. They have therefore set up standards for continuing professional development and have published *Guidance on Continuing Professional Development*, which you can view online at www.gmc-uk.org/education/continuing_professional_development/cpd_guidance.asp. This sets out the principles on which CPD should be based and the roles of the relevant organisations involved in its delivery and quality assurance.

All doctors working in the NHS including trainees are required to maintain a portfolio of evidence of their performance as a basis for their appraisals. They are able to use existing educational processes and documentation, thus theoretically no extra effort should be required to maintain the portfolio. It is based on the consultant form that is, in turn, designed around *Good Medical Practice* (GMC 2006) that can be accessed online at www.gmc.uk.org/guidance/good_medical_practice/probity/financial_and_commercial_dealings.asp. Details of the requirements of the form can be found on the Department of Health website: www.dh.gov.uk/assetRoot/04/08/03/27/04080327.doc. Most royal colleges and specialty bodies now have their own dedicated paperwork, documents, guidance and specialty-related forms to assist.

Registration arrangements with the GMC have also changed. Graduates from UK medical schools are required for the first 12 months to work in an 'approved (by the GMC) practice setting'. You can find out more about this online at www.gmc-uk.org/doctors/registration_news/new_framework/approved_practice_settings.asp. After you have completed 12 months in an approved practice setting, if you can provide evidence of satisfactory performance, you are eligible to apply for 'release from the requirement to work in approved practice setting'. You can access material on this online at www.gmc-uk.org/doctors/registration_applications/release_from_aps/release_from_aps_p1.asp.

Once registered, you have to continue to be 'fit to practice' as set out in the GMC's *Good Medical Practice*. This is sent to every doctor, although you can read and download a copy online at the GMC website.

You are also required to:
- pay an annual retention fee (ARF) (there is a lower-income discount)
- provide a registered postal address
- tell the GMC anything that might affect your registration, a change of name for example
- make your seven-digit GMC number available to patients and on prescriptions.

If you leave the UK and ask to have your name taken off the register, your application for restoration may be referred to a Committee of the GMC, who will decide whether your registration can be restored. In certain circumstances they may request certificates of good standing relating to any period more than five years ago and make further inquiries as appropriate, or require you to resubmit your original primary medical qualification(s).

If you relinquish your registration you can still use the title 'doctor' but cannot claim to be a registered medical practitioner. You can act as a 'Good Samaritan' to someone in an emergency and are not liable for the ARF.

Doctors in training will have to participate in revalidation (*see* p. 51). But the intention is that doctors in training should be able to use the record of their progress through training for the purposes of their revalidation. It is not anticipated that trainees should have to meet a separate set of requirements.

Assessment

I have already drawn your attention to the sometimes confused and sometimes slack use of terminology so I will continue to draw your attention to alternative names given for various processes. Essentially, assessment is a judgement or measurement of your achievements. It requires some method for measurement and being work-based is inevitably based on work-placed tasks. The 'Gold Guide' defines assessment as a formally defined process within the curriculum in which a trainee's progress in the training programme is assessed and measured using a range of defined and validated assessment tools, along with professional and triangulated judgements about the trainee's rate of progress. It results in an 'outcome' following evaluation of the written evidence of progress and is essential if the trainee is to progress and able to confirm that the required competences are being achieved. (*See* www.mmc.nhs.uk/specialty_training _2010/gold_guide.aspx.)

Formative assessment

There are two types of assessment: formative and summative.

'Formative' or 'educational' assessment is also known as 'appraisal', so feedback on appraisal of performance is an educational process and hence a formative assessment. It is focused on the learner and their educational needs. It attempts to measure skills, behaviours, attitudes or knowledge. Being assessed enables you to identify gaps and structure your educational plans. Finding weaknesses ought to be encouraged, as it provides for learning opportunities. A trainee should have a learning plan agreed through negotiation and openness, not coercion or manipulation.

Summative assessment

'Summative' assessment attempts to measure ability; for example, to permit progress over a performance hurdle such as in the annual assessment of specialist trainees. The first significant formalised summative assessment integrated into medical training was introduced in 1997 with the Calman reforms, with the record of individual in-training assessment (RITA).

Annual Review of Competence Progression

The Annual Review of Competence Progression (ARCP) has replaced RITA. The ARCP provides for the overall assessment of progress from evidence which trainees are required to supply, as well as the structured report written by the trainee's educational supervisor. This is a report that the trainee and supervisor ought to have agreed on and should reflect the learning agreement for the period under review.

It shows the results of in-work assessments, examinations and further activities required by the specialty curriculum (e.g. logbooks, publications, audits). The PMETB's document *Workplace Based Assessment: a guide for implementation* (2009) provides detailed guidance on this process and the medical colleges and specialty groups all have advice and guidance on their websites.

This report then provides the summary of the assessment evidence for the annual review process. The outcome from the annual review provides the evidence for the appraisal process designed to reassure employers that the performance of doctors in postgraduate specialty training is satisfactory.

The ARCP then produces a report that contributes to the trainee's further educational appraisal and forms the basis of the trainee's workplace-based (NHS) appraisal. The educational supervisor has a duty to alert the medical director to any areas of concern raised by the ARCP regarding the trainee's performance in the workplace.

Summative assessment also tests for skills, behaviours, attitudes and knowledge, such as the methods outlined below under Modernising Medical Careers. Another aim of summative assessment is to identify trainees who are not ready for independent practice as well as confirming those who are ready. The results of summative assessment are not confidential and outcomes can affect career progression.

Modes of assessment

Nationally standardised modes of assessment have been introduced as part of MMC and include the following.

o **MSF (multisource feedback)** of which there are two versions:
  ‣ **Mini-PAT (mini-peer assessment tool):** the trainee nominates eight assessors from among clinical colleagues, who fill out questionnaires; together with the trainee's self-assessment these are electronically collated and fed back through an educational supervisor.
  ‣ **TAB (team assessment behaviour)** or **360-degree feedback** (*see* p. 53): a form is completed by 10, mainly clinical, co-workers. This too is summarised and fed back by an educational supervisor and included in the trainee's portfolio.
o **Mini–CEX (clinical evaluation exercise):** this is a 15-minute snapshot of a doctor–patient interaction. It is designed to assess the clinical skills, attitudes and behaviours of the trainee. Six of these are undertaken each year, with a different observer for each encounter.
o **DOPS (direct observation of procedural skills):** trainees are required to undertake six different procedures under observation. An assessor can be any appropriate clinician who is selected by the trainee.
o **CbD (case-based discussion):** the trainee selects two case records from patients

they have recently seen and in whose notes they have made an entry. The assessor selects one of these for discussion with the trainee. The purpose is to assess clinical decision making and the application of medical knowledge in the care of the trainee's own patients.

Modernising Medical Careers (MMC)

Since 2003, medical education and training in the UK has been going through radical reform under the MMC programme. A new Foundation Programme for medical school graduates started in 2005, followed by new specialty and GP training programmes in 2007. For details of specialty training, see the MMC website at www. mmc.nhs.uk/default.aspx or Google 'Gold Guide', where you will find information on applying for specialty training posts in the NHS in England, as well as information on changes to the recruitment and training process. There are links to information on MMC in the other countries of the UK: Wales (at www.mmcwales.org), Scotland (at www.mmc.scot.nhs.uk) and Northern Ireland (at www.nimdta.gov.uk).

Beginning with the Foundation Programme, two years of training occur between medical school and specialty or general practice training. During this period trainees have the opportunity to gain experience in a series of placements in a variety of specialties. The first year (F1) builds upon the knowledge, skills and competences acquired in undergraduate training. The F2 year continues with the focus on assessment and management of the acutely ill patient. Training also encompasses the generic professional skills applicable to all areas of medicine – teamwork, time management, communication and IT skills. From the Foundation Programme's website (www.foundation programme.nhs.uk) you can download a number of useful related documents and a handbook for Foundation applicants.

MMC tries to provide consistent national standards for training through better-structured and managed programmes with competency-based curricula approved by the independent Postgraduate Medical Education and Training Board. PMETB was created in 2005 to set the criteria and standards for training, including approving the curricula for the programmes and taking over these functions from the Specialist Training Authority (STA) and the Joint Committee on Postgraduate Training for General Practice (JCPTGP).

PMETB's aim is to have a higher proportion of patient care delivered by an appropriately skilled workforce. For trainees, the new programmes' structures attempt to provide high-quality training, better formal supervision and continuous development of acquired competencies, backed up by good evidence.

The deaneries are responsible for the management and delivery of postgraduate medical education and for the continuing professional development of all doctors and dentists. This includes ensuring that all training posts provide the necessary opportunities for doctors and dentists in training to realise their full potential and provide high-quality patient care. The deaneries are also responsible for trainers, educational supervisors and educational leaders, their training needs and educational development.

NHS Medical Education England (MEE)

A new advisory body established in January 2009 was set up in response to a recommendation from the Tooke review (the MMC Inquiry that reported in 2008) and operates at arm's length from Ministers. The full title is 'Aspiring to Excellence: Findings and Final Recommendations of the Independent Inquiry into Modernising Medical Careers'.

The Inquiry into Modernising Medical Schools was led by Professor Sir John Tooke, Chair of the Medical Schools Council. There was also an interim report published in November 2007, following an extensive consultation with almost 40 000 responses; the final report of the Inquiry was published in 2008. Recommendations include the proposal for a new co-ordinating body, NHS: Medical Education England (MEE).

MEE provides independent expert advice on training and education for doctors, dentists, healthcare scientists and pharmacists. It also oversees the development of training programmes, including modular training and modular credentialing that open up the possibilities for flexibility. Modular credentialing – formal accreditation at defined points – is attempting to make it easier for people to move in and out of training, move between programmes and gain a wide range of experience.

So who are the key figures in this new structure? Below I attempt to provide a summary with their main roles. Their roles and responsibilities are pretty much standard, although there is some marginal variation within deaneries and trusts. Three significant roles are identified in the MMC process – these had existed previously under similar titles but often with differing or unclear role descriptions. The UK National Association of Clinical Tutors (NACT) in 2009 defined their roles and much of the information below is based on their descriptions with additional material from various colleges and specialty opinions.

Clinical supervisor

There must be at least one named clinical supervisor in each training placement. They are the doctor responsible for making sure trainees receive appropriate training and experience to meet the objectives outlined in their Personal Development Plan. They are also responsible for deciding whether individual placements have been completed. Being responsible for teaching and supervising trainees, they would normally be expected to work with the trainee for at least part of their rotation and be involved with assessments.

Their responsibilities would include the following.

o Supervise day-to-day clinical and professional practice.
o Support the assessment process.
o Arrange a work programme to enable the trainee to attend fixed educational sessions.
o Contribute to feedback to trainee.
o Contribute to feedback to trainee's educational supervisor.
o Facilitate trainee's acquisition of new skills in accordance with learning plan.
o Facilitate trainee's acquisition of new knowledge in accordance with learning plan.
o Ensure trainee has competence to fulfil requirements of post.

o Ensure primary care trust clinical governance structures are adhered to.
o Ensure primary care trust work policies are adhered to (health, holidays and study leave).
o Attend training and update sessions in clinical supervision and assessment tools.
o Complete assessment tools.
o Oversee the clinical performance and progress of a named trainee.
o Meet away from the clinical area regularly (minimum one hour per week) to discuss cases, provide feedback and monitor progress of learning objectives.
o Ensure those in clinical team provide appropriate clinical supervision and understand the relevant workplace assessments.

Educational supervisor

The educational supervisor is the doctor responsible for making sure that the trainee receives appropriate training and experience through developing clear objectives based on the relevant specialty curriculum. They decide whether agreed competencies have been successfully achieved in individual placements. The educational supervisor is responsible through the Postgraduate Dean's educational contract both for educational and workplace-based appraisal of the trainee.

The clinical supervisor and educational supervisor could be the same person or two people. It is common for Foundation Programme trainees to have the same educational supervisor throughout the two years of the programme and who doesn't normally work with the trainee. The educational supervisor should work closely with the Clinical Tutor/Foundation Programme Tutor.

The educational supervisor's responsibilities include the following.
o Be responsible for a named trainee for all aspects of personal and professional development and progress through the programme.
o Perform regular educational and annual NHS appraisal.
o Attend educational meetings and completing reports, involved in ARCP/RITA, and may also help in recruitment.
o Involvement in careers guidance and with trainees in difficulty.
o Help to define a trainee's learning needs.
o Help to formulate trainee's personal development plan.
o Ensure that the trainee understands and engages in the assessment process.
o Identify and facilitate areas needing development.
o Provide support to the trainee for the development and review of their Learning Portfolio.
o Provide feedback on trainee progress – both clinical and non-clinical activity.
o Ensure that appropriate training opportunities are made available to learn and gain the required competences.
o Ensure that trainees whom they supervise maintain appropriate records of assessment.
o Meet on a regular basis, ideally three meetings per attachment – beginning, mid-point and end.
o Maintain proper records of supervision meetings.

○ Complete required documentation in relation to the learning portfolio.
○ Regular formative appraisal but not normally assessments.
○ Be the first point of contact for the trainee who has concerns/issues about their training.
○ Contact the relevant Foundation Training Programme Directors (FTPD) should the level of performance of any foundation trainee give rise for concern.
○ Provide mentoring support, or know how to access it.
○ Identify a trainee in difficulty and source means of relevant support.
○ Maintain proper records of action plan agreed for trainee in difficulty.
○ Provide career guidance and support.
○ Attend educational supervisor training course and ensure commitment to updating supervisory skills.

As a trainee you would normally expect the following.
○ A meeting with your educational supervisor at the start of each hospital placement.
○ An induction meeting with clinical supervisor within one week.
○ Perhaps a meeting midway in placement.
○ The final review of each hospital placement.

Foundation Training Programme Director

Once again we are in difficulty with definitions, not only between deaneries, but also between the four NHS organisations in the devolved UK. The Foundation Training Programme Director or Foundation Programme Tutor is the individual appointed by the deanery and trust to manage and lead a foundation training programme. At Foundation Programme (FP) level this is the person responsible for organising and providing quality assurance of the FP training in a trust. They also help to develop, maintain and improve trust Foundation Programmes, oversee and monitor the FP generic skills programme and ensure that all FP trainees receive appropriate coaching. They manage Foundation training programmes across a locality-based group of local education providers on behalf of the deanery-based Foundation School. The Programme Directors:
○ organise the posts within a programme
○ organise the teaching
○ identify the educational supervisor for each FP trainee
○ are responsible for the delivery of the faculty development programme for foundation programme trainers and assessors.

You can find out more about the Foundation Programme at their website (www. foundationprogramme.nhs.uk/pages/home).

Trainers

○ Supervise/coach trainees on ward rounds, in clinic, in operative lists and out of hours.

o   Undertake a small number per year of workplace-based assessments (fewer than 10 a year).
o   Contribute to 360-degree feedback.

Clinical Tutor (Director of Medical Education)

The Clinical Tutor, in some trusts also known as Director of Medical Education, is the individual appointed by the Postgraduate Dean and the trust to manage postgraduate medical education within the trust. It is their responsibility on behalf of the Dean to ensure that the learning environment within the trust supports the provision of high-quality postgraduate medical education and training. They provide professional leadership and vision for the organisation on medical education issues and work closely with the Postgraduate Dean and foundation school to develop the team of consultants and other health professionals who are responsible for supporting elements of the Foundation Programme as well as the provision of specialty training. The Clinical Tutor's role is to:

o   support Educational Supervisors and Tutors with trainees in difficulty and provide pastoral and career support to trainees as necessary
o   manage the Postgraduate Centre
o   administer study leave
o   maintain and develop the profile of medical education within local education provider (LEP)
o   ensure delivery of the Education Contract
o   ensure quality control of all postgraduate medical education (PGME) training programmes.

Specialty College Tutor

Role varies from college to college but they are responsible via the relevant Training Programme to the Director and Chair of the Deanery Regional Specialty Training Committee (STC) and to the Postgraduate Dean for co-ordinating postgraduate training and assessment.

They have to undergo instruction as prescribed by the specialty body or college and thereafter assign trainees to educational supervisors. The Specialty College Tutor's role is to:

o   co-ordinate formative assessments of trainees
o   arrange induction programmes for new trainees
o   meet regularly with and advise trainees within specialty
o   maintain an environment within a department or multi-professional team that supports training and delivers the curriculum and relevant assessments
o   support trainees and trainers
o   attend department and trust education committees
o   attend Deanery STC if necessary
o   ensure systems are in place for specialty induction, quality control of training provided, formal education delivery and study leave management
o   be involved in careers guidance and with trainees in difficulty.

Training Programme Director

The Programme Director has responsibility for allocation of training posts, supervision of programmes of training, regular formal assessment, problem solving and feedback on progress. They manage the delivery of the programme of specialist training to the standards set by their college and now PMETB. They use the resources provided by the Postgraduate Dean with whom lies the responsibility for appointment and indemnity and to whom they are legally accountable. The distribution of tasks and responsibilities between individuals in key roles varies even within one deanery, influenced by the local custom, the specialty and the number of trainees involved.

The Training Programme Director is also responsible for:

○ management of and participation in the appointments process
○ management of the programme generally, of curriculum delivery
○ provision of appropriate training programmes for doctors with differing needs
○ management of the appraisal and assessment processes for trainees and jointly with the STC Chair for Quality Assurance of the programme (i.e. educational opportunities, trainers, etc)
○ curriculum design, based on the appropriate Royal College Syllabus/Curriculum and PMETB requirements
○ careers information and advice and support for doctors/dentists who get into difficulty.

Specialist Training Committee Chair

The deanery STCs identified with each Certificate of Completion of Specialist Training (CCST)-defined specialty are the key committees for implementing the specialist training programmes, for purposes of:

○ good management
○ appropriate accountability
○ secure indemnity.

These STCs must not only be 'deanery-based' but deanery-appointed in collaboration with their college or faculty – taking account of local views and fair 'balance'. The Chair oversees on behalf of the deanery the activity and proper functioning of the STC, liaising as necessary with the relevant college, faculty or staff advisory committee (SAC), and supports the programme director(s). The Chair needs to be legally accountable to the deanery (*see* annex 3 and 4 of 'Green CoPMED book') regarding indemnity that is highly relevant. This requirement for indemnity applies to all those holding lead roles or who take part in appointment or assessment processes.

Chairs of STCs, and programme directors, are at the same time professionally accountable to their college or faculty. No job description is available but an important document in relation to this role is the 'Green CoPMED book': *A Guide to the Management and Quality Assurance of Postgraduate Medical and Dental Education*, which can be downloaded from www.docstoc.com/docs/3424768/academy-of-medical-royal-colleges-COPMeD-UK.

Regional Advisor and Deputy Regional Advisor

Appointed by their college after consultation with the deanery and the relevant specialty advisers and consultants, they represent their college in relation to the specialty or a group of specialties in a number of roles. Most 'role descriptions' include education and training and many include the vetting of proposed consultant posts and non-consultant career posts and advising the NHS (regional offices, health authorities or trusts) and deanery on other matters relating to their specialty.

They will always play a major part in the work of their deanery STC, and may or may not chair that committee: there is a range of college and deanery preferences in this matter based on professional and geographical factors and the number of trainees involved. Responsibilities vary between colleges.

College websites

Some colleges have set up websites to assist their trainees; for example, the Intercollegiate Surgical Curriculum Programme (ISCP) website (www.iscp.ac.uk). This site houses the curriculum for the nine surgical specialties and, in a secure area, trainees' electronic portfolios and the learning agreements that support training. All trainees using the new curriculum need to register as indeed do consultants and other professionals who will be training, assessing and supervising training. It is a convenient way to assess your syllabus and logbooks.

Variations in appraisal across the UK

The Royal College of General Practitioners published a guide to *The Principles of GP Appraisal* (RCGP 2008) with a lot of useful information. Some 82% of GPs in the UK work in England, 10% work in Scotland, 5% in Wales and 3% in Northern Ireland. Deaneries in Wales, Scotland and Northern Ireland have been actively engaged in GP appraisal. There has been involvement of CPD tutors in Scotland, Wales and Northern Ireland in their national GP appraisal schemes. Deaneries appear to be involved in the GP appraisal process through:

o the quality assurance process (Scotland, NI, Wales)
o training GP appraisers (Scotland, NI, Wales, although in England some external consultants are used)
o providing ongoing development for GP appraisers
o delivery of GP appraisal (e.g. in Wales and Northern Ireland deanery teams have been commissioned to run the whole process on behalf of primary care organisations)
o evaluation of the appraisal process and of appraiser performance
o education by assessing GP learning needs and providing related educational support
o investigation and clarification of concerns relating to the performance of appraisees.

GP appraisal in England

Responsibility for implementing GP appraisal rests with the primary care trusts (PCTs). The outcomes of GP appraisals are generally fed back to the PCTs, and inform PCTs about the educational needs of GPs locally. Where there are GP tutors employed by the deanery, this information may be shared with them. Some deaneries are engaged in the quality assurance of GP appraisal in partnership with PCTs. Currently, appraisal is often regarded as purely developmental (formative or educational) and seen by some to be no more than a 'cosy chat' between professionals.

GP appraisal in Scotland

NHS Education for Scotland (NES) has overall responsibility for GP appraisal. Working with the Royal College of General Practitioners (RCGP) and others (NES) has developed and implemented appraisal in Scotland. NES has undertaken quantitative and qualitative research into the influence of appraisal and research has also looked at the training undertaken by appraisers. Although employed locally, appraisers are a central team and are responsible for selection and training and the provision of the resources to support appraisal.

External quality assurance of the scheme is being carried out by Quality Improvement Scotland and there is an ongoing system of internal quality assurance. NES is responsible for the IT systems to support appraisal. The Scottish appraisal website has undergone extensive development and a long-term aim is to link with e-portfolio.

Scotland is currently examining how the amount of objective evidence presented at appraisal can be increased and a national evaluation project of peer-reviewed evidence has begun.

GP appraisal in Wales

In 2003 the National Assembly agreed a Service Level Agreement with the Wales Deanery to roll out the GP appraisal programme based on the preceding Welsh pilot scheme. The appraisers are selected, appointed, trained and paid by the deanery. The deanery works with PCOs to develop the appraisal process so that it is relevant to clinical governance systems.

A computerised database is maintained from which to access anonymised needs declared in GPs' personal development plans (PDPs). Information is collated to support CPD and to identify local constraints.

The Wales Deanery's appraisal system has an integrated quality management process which includes external quality assurance activity. Among numerous other projects, minimum evidence sets for appraisal are being developed. The deanery is working with the GMC to define and test systems of appraisal and clinical governance.

GP appraisal in Northern Ireland

In Northern Ireland the NI Medical and Dental Training Agency (NIMDTA) has a service level agreement to manage the GP appraisal process for each of the four health and social service boards and is accountable to a Central Board of Management which has representation from the Department of Health, Social Services and Public Safety (DHSSPS), RCGP, Northern Ireland General Practitioners Committee (NIGPC) and NIMDTA.

The Agency recruits, trains and employs the appraisers (on the GP Educator pay scale) and manages the whole process.

There are communication protocols and close links with the four boards, particularly in relation to the Performers' List. There are also close links with the NI GP Education Consortium, which represents all GP Education providers.

Learning needs identified from GPs' personal development plans are collated and forwarded to the Consortium for action.

GPs can choose any of the appraisers employed by NIMDTA. There is an online system for booking appraisals. Appraisees must choose a different appraiser after three years.

Basic principles of appraisal and assessment

o Doctors will require training in the skills necessary to assess or appraise others.
o Doctors may also require training in how to prepare and make the most of the experience.
o From the outside it should be agreed whether the meeting is confidential or not.
o Those involved must know which type of process is being carried out.
o Should a change be required (assessment moving into personal counselling), agreement is necessary.
o There must be mutual trust based on fairness and objectivity.
o Some types, summative and formative (educational or appraisal) assessment, do not sit easily together, although it is inevitable with trainees that some overlap might occur.

Managing the appraisal process

Preparation for appraisal relies heavily on the appraisee, who should have collected information about their performance from a range of sources, including:
o patients (e.g. through a patient survey)
o close colleagues such as partners or other professionals (e.g. through a peer-associate questionnaire)
o managers, where appropriate
o colleagues who refer to, or accept, referrals from the doctor
o the doctor (e.g. through a self-assessment questionnaire).

It may be that 360-degree feedback is available, in which case this is likely to provide the simplest and most reliable means of collecting information.

The main aim of this section is to provide a basis for successful medical appraisal interviews. Appraisal is an integral part of specialist registrar (SpR) training and has become a mandatory element in the revalidation process. Although the purpose of this book does not specifically require covering consultant appraisal for revalidation, the principles and suggested practice outlined below apply equally to most appraisal situations.

Trainee appraisal is essentially a formative process. Although some judgement is involved it is normally intended that the trainee should be developed rather than assessed. Appraisal is intended to be part of the educational process. Kolb *et al.* (1984) proposed a model of learning which I explored in Chapter 1 (*see* Figure 1.2).

A well-conducted appraisal meeting provides an opportunity for the trainee to gain important new experience through interaction with a senior colleague whose opinion is important to the trainee. The appraiser helps the trainee to reflect on experience and also assists in the acquisition and development of understanding of new concepts. It remains for the trainee to go out and test the learning in their own way, taking risks (under the supervision of a senior colleague) and acquiring new experience to be reflected upon later.

Appraisal can:
○ help identify educational needs at an early stage
○ assist in the skills of self-reflection and self-appraisal that will be needed through-out a trainee's career
○ enable learning opportunities that will be helpful to the trainee to be provided quickly
○ provide a mechanism for reviewing progress and identifying problems in time for remedial action to be taken
○ provide a mechanism for giving feedback on the quality of training provided
○ make training more efficient and effective.

Appraisal meetings should take place at the beginning, halfway through and at the end of the post. The first meeting sets up the training agreement which describes the learning objectives and confirms the support needed by the trainee during their time in the post. It is important that the trainee comes properly prepared for this meeting and guidelines for this are given below. The second meeting is primarily concerned with reviewing progress, designing new learning opportunities if they are required and revising learning goals. The final meeting again reviews the trainee's experience, assists the trainee to reflect on experience gained, and helps to make sense of the complexities of the learning process. It will also, if required, address career-related issues. Appraisers should seek feedback from their trainees on the training and appraisal process at the end of every appraisal meeting.

Preparation for the appraisal meeting
As indicated earlier, in your current role you may, at different times, be both appraiser and appraisee. First, I address the process for the appraisee.

Preparation: the trainee
You should be aware that the success of the appraisal meeting depends on adequate preparation by both parties. The list under 'Preparing the agenda' (*see* p. 47) should help you to determine your most important topics. You should ask yourself the following questions, and take notes to the meeting.

Work performance
○ Which areas of the work do you enjoy most?

○ Which tasks do you feel you perform the best?
○ Which areas do you find most challenging and why?
○ How might you have improved your performance?

Skills/abilities
○ Reflect on your strengths and weaknesses.
○ Which skills do you have which you believe are well developed?
○ Identify those skills which need more development.

Learning objectives
○ What learning objectives would you like to agree for the coming period of training?

Training
○ Are there any specific training courses, or areas of need, which you would like to have addressed in the coming period?

Career
○ What are the main career-related issues facing you at present? Are there still key decisions to be made? What help do you need with them?

Preparation: the appraiser

In your work as an SpR and, more significantly, as a consultant, you are likely to be called upon to appraise colleagues. I concentrate here on the appraisal of trainees rather than colleagues. The aims of a trainee appraisal meeting are to identify relevant learning goals, to agree and commit to them, to reflect on and make sense of the trainee's past experience and to agree and record actions based on the discussion. These might be for either the appraiser or trainee to implement.

The following guidelines are intended to enhance the quality of the appraisal for both parties.

○ **Plan the meeting**. Dates and times for all meetings to be held during the post should be determined well in advance.
○ **The trainee should be helped to prepare for the meeting**. After you have prepared an agenda you should show it to the trainee. The trainee preparation guidelines could be given to the trainee and discussed a few days before the meeting.
○ **Relevant materials**. The curriculum, timetable, job description, rotas, previous appraisal records and notes of feedback from third parties should be collected together and considered before the meeting.
○ **Suitable venue**. A quiet room guaranteed free from interruptions should be used. Bleeps and mobile phones *must always* be switched off or passed to a colleague.
○ **Sufficient time**. There is no 'correct' amount of time to set aside for an appraisal meeting, but it is unlikely that much will be achieved in under half an hour. Note that the appraisal must take place in protected time.
○ **Third parties**. Discuss the trainee with other consultants, trainees, nurses, midwives, technicians, physiotherapists or others as necessary to gain a rounded picture of the trainee.

Preparing the agenda

It helps if the pattern of the meeting is clear from the beginning for both parties. An agenda should be prepared and shared before the meeting. The following checklist should help you to prepare and conduct the appraisal. Choose from it the items you consider should make up the agenda for the meeting.

○ **Education**. What, if any, examinations should be in preparation? What courses should be undertaken?

○ **Academic/research**. Is advice necessary on research projects, or decisions to be made regarding suitable research designs?

○ **Clinical experience and skills**. What specified procedures does the curriculum indicate? What levels of understanding and competence are indicated? Is good manual dexterity and hand/eye co-ordination necessary? Is experience of clinical risk management a requirement?

○ **Knowledge**. What is an appropriate level of clinical knowledge? Is knowledge or use of evidence-based practice a requirement?

○ **Organisation and planning**. What level of ability to organise their own work and self-organisation are demanded of the trainee? Is active participation in audit an element of the training at this stage?

○ **Teaching skills**. Should the trainee be gaining experience of teaching others and, if so, at what level?

○ **Career**. Should the trainee be helped to make career decisions at this stage? What help may be necessary? Would sharing your own experience be helpful to the trainee?

○ **Personal skills and attributes**. The wide range of personal skills demanded in the work of a doctor is indicated below. Select those you feel should be discussed with the trainee.

▶ *Interpersonal communication:* rapport building, listening, empathising, persuading and negotiating skills.

▶ *Decisiveness:* taking responsibility, exerting appropriate authority.

▶ *Team working:* co-operating with others, leading as required, seeking guidance.

▶ *Flexibility and resilience:* able to adapt to rapidly changing circumstances and cope with setbacks.

▶ *Thoroughness:* well-prepared, self-disciplined, punctual and committed to carry tasks through to completion.

▶ *Drive and enthusiasm:* committed to patients and colleagues, motivated to achieve, curious, displaying initiative.

▶ *Self-managed learning:* takes learning opportunities, reflects on experience, seeks guidance and advice.

▶ *Probity:* honest, showing integrity and awareness of ethical dilemmas.

○ Feedback from the trainee is usually helpful in enabling you to improve your approach.

Finally, the outcomes of the meeting should be recorded. It helps to remind you to include this stage by noting it in the agenda.

Conducting an appraisal meeting

The pattern of the meeting, partly determined by the level and experience of the trainee, should be dictated by the trainee's needs. Effective appraisal means getting the trainee to identify strengths and areas of need and to propose ways of meeting the latter. Although guided by the appraiser, a successful meeting will feel as if it has been led by the trainee's priorities.

Confirm the agenda

The agenda should have been determined in advance with the trainee's help, but it is worthwhile briefly re-establishing the aims and key items for discussion. If a record of the previous appraisal is available, this should be used to inform the discussion at this stage.

Review past performance

Get the trainee talking as soon as possible. Use questions to open up issues and probe to help the trainee to explore their own strengths and weaknesses in the light of their performance. Try to avoid being directive. Allow the trainee to describe their perspective on issues and help them to reflect by using open and probing questions. Focus on specific aspects of the work. Give positive feedback where possible, particularly as a balance to any comments on less successful aspects of the trainee's work. Giving feedback requires a high level of skill and sensitivity. It demands a careful blend of drawing out the trainee to describe their own strengths and particularly weaknesses. Be direct in explaining concerns that you have and that the trainee does not appear to recognise.

Explore and agree current learning needs

The trainee should have identified key learning needs in advance, but these may need to be modified in the light of the previous discussion. It may also be affected by information you have obtained from third parties in preparation for the meeting. You should remember that the responsibility for the trainee's learning is a joint one. Avoid taking on a list of jobs which could be more suitably undertaken by the trainee. Make brief notes to ensure you can recall critical issues. Reflect on learning objectives agreed for the post.

Agree learning objectives for the next period

These should be 'SMART'. This means they should be:

o **S**pecific – relate to specific tasks and activities not general statements about improvement
o **M**easurable – it should be possible to assess whether or not it has been achieved
o **A**ttainable – given the time available it should be possible for the trainee to achieve the desired outcome
o **R**ealistic – set within the trainee's capability
o **T**imed – the next appraisal date or earlier should be agreed as the time for reviewing the achievement of the objective.

Review and record decisions

You may wish to make brief notes throughout the meeting in order to ensure that all the key points are reviewed at the end. It is vital that a record is kept of the outcome of the meeting. This should be agreed at the end of the meeting and a copy kept by both parties. It will prove useful at the next meeting and may also form a useful document for the trainee to use as a record of progress in a logbook or portfolio. Doctors should retain records of appraisal meetings for their revalidation folders.

Get feedback on your performance

It is not common for appraisers to welcome informal feedback from the trainee at the end of an appraisal meeting. Indeed, it could prove to be an uncomfortable experience. Nevertheless, if the relationship between the two has developed positively it can be very helpful for the appraiser to get an immediate indication of the benefits gained by the trainee. Bolder trainees may even give constructive criticism of the training received and any weaknesses perceived by them in the scheme. While this may be difficult it will help future trainees and give the appraiser greater satisfaction in the long term. Alternatives include written feedback forms, which College tutors often use to route feedback to the Royal College.

Dealing with difficult issues

Confidentiality

There are mixed messages from some sources regarding the confidential nature of the appraisal meeting. Typically, it is suggested that if trainees are to feel free to express concerns about their capability or commitment to a specialty, the appraiser must indicate that he or she will maintain confidentiality. On the other hand, in some cases the appraiser is also the assessor who is required to complete an assessment, in the case of SpRs for the Record of Individual (In-training) Training Assessment. The final appraisal of F1 trainees is intended as the indicator of suitability for registration. In these and other cases, the appraiser/assessor is in a difficult situation if confidentiality is an issue. There may also be circumstances when the appraiser feels that in the interests of patient safety information about the trainee should be passed on to others. Appraisers should help trainees to recognise that confidentiality is limited by the above conditions and that they will do all they can to support the trainee while ensuring that the normal procedures are followed.

Conflict

The management of conflict is addressed in Chapter 4. Disagreements are bound to arise from time to time and these should be resolved quickly to avoid escalation. Should serious conflict arise between an appraiser and trainee it serves little purpose to attempt to resolve it since the trainee will always be concerned that fair assessment is compromised. A new appraiser should be found as quickly as possible.

Serious personal problems

Difficulties in appraisal may arise due to the serious nature of personal problems that afflict some trainees from time to time. It is important that the appraiser takes responsibility for ensuring the trainee receives suitable support in these circumstances. They should not, however, assume responsibility for taking on a counselling role or becoming personally burdened with the trainee's situation.

Further advice on counselling is given below. Occupational health officers or personnel departments can usually assist in such circumstances.

Lack of personal insight

Occasionally, trainees seem to lack the ability to see their own weaknesses as others see them. This can be particularly true where there is a lack of interpersonal skill. It may also be that trainees are not able to see their lack of progress in developing clinical competence and judgement. It is important to distinguish between those who really are unaware of the negative impact they create or the concerns of other staff at the inadequacy of their clinical practice and those who refuse to admit to weakness in order to protect themselves from negative consequences. In the latter case it is important to help the trainee to recognise the value of talking about their problems since it may lead to better career decisions if they are struggling with the demands of the specialty in which they are working. Once again, the most helpful way to do this is to use open and probing questions focused on specific examples of their performance to get them to confront the problem. Those trainees who truly are unable to see their weakness even after supportive questioning and gentle challenge will only perhaps come to terms with their situation when they fail an assessment. It is crucial that the clinical tutor and perhaps the Postgraduate Dean is made aware of such problems at as early a stage in training as possible.

White paper 'Trust, Assurance and Safety: the regulation of health professionals in the 21st century' (2007)

This paper contains the first definitive statement for relicensing, as in future all doctors will require a licence to practise that enables them to remain on the medical register. It will need to be renewed every five years. In order to bring objective assurance of continuing fitness to practise, the appraisal process would include 'summative' elements that confirm that a doctor has objectively met the standards expected.

Specialist recertification would apply to all specialists, including GPs, requiring them to demonstrate they meet the standards that apply to their medical specialty, which would be set and assessed by the medical royal colleges, their specialist societies and approved by the GMC.

It also made clear that the appraisal process would be a central component of revalidation and would be both formative and summative to ensure that the required standards were met. Within the English NHS, information gathered under the 'Knowledge and Skills Framework' would be used as far as possible as the basis of revalidation with any additional requirements justified by risk analysis.

The full text is available at www.official-documents.gov.uk/document/cm70/7013/7013.pdf.

The White Paper indicated that Scotland, Wales and Northern Ireland would need to consider how they wished to take this forward within their particular contexts. It is not possible within the limitations of this book to outline differences but merely to emphasise that essentially they are very similar. Appraisal paperwork for each country has been individualised. In England the responsibility for implementing GP appraisal is with PCTs, whereas in Scotland the NHS Education for Scotland has overall responsibility. The system for GPs has been set up with help from the Scottish General Practitioners Committee (SGPC), Royal College of General Practitioners in Scotland (RCGP Scotland) and Scottish Executive Health Department (SEHD). In Northern Ireland it is the responsibility of Local Health and Social Care Groups.

NHS Employers (*see* Part 2, Chapter 1 on understanding the NHS) was pleased that employers' views had helped shape the White Paper, saying that it recognised the importance of local employers in professional regulation and gave them new responsibilities to confirm the continuing competency of their staff for revalidation purposes. The proposals that would affect employers were as follows:

- all health professionals will be required to undergo periodic revalidation based on appraisal
- the introduction of a system of regional GMC affiliates who would provide support for local employers in addressing concerns about doctors and assuring local revalidation processes a new measure of recorded concerns to allow for the local regulation of concerns about a doctor's conduct or practice
- closer co-ordination between employers and regulators when a health professional enters employment for the first time.

NHS Employers believed that the proposals likely to have the most impact upon employers include:

- better support available for patients who want to register concerns
- all organisations providing services to NHS patients to have clear policies setting out how staff can raise concerns
- more rigorous checks on references and qualifications when health professionals are recruited
- improving the way information about professionals from different sources is handled so that appropriate action can be taken
- primary care organisations adopting best practice in investigating and acting on concerns
- in addition there would be new responsibilities for PCTs for handling complaints against GPs.

Licensing and revalidation

Revalidation is the process that combines relicensing and recertification. Revalidation for UK doctors was originally proposed in 1975, but it was not until 1998 and the

Bristol Inquiry that there was any impetus to implement this idea. In November 2009 the GMC introduced the licence to practise. All doctors are required by law to hold both registration and a licence to practise whether full-time, part-time, as a locum, privately, in the NHS, employed or self-employed.

After licensing, however, recertification is set to start in 2010. This will be added as part of system called revalidation and will require doctors to renew their licence periodically. Revalidation is to be the process by which doctors will demonstrate to the GMC on a regular basis that they remain up to date and fit to practise; it will involve three elements:

o   to confirm that a licensed doctor's practice is in accordance with the GMC's generic standards
o   to confirm that doctors on the GMC's specialist register or GP register continue to meet the standards appropriate for their specialty
o   to identify, for further investigation and remediation, poor practice where local systems are not robust enough to do this or do not exist.

The UK Revalidation Programme Board has been formed to oversee the practical delivery of medical revalidation across the four countries in the UK.

Surveys and polls on doctors.net.uk show that there is scepticism about the agenda and motivation behind this process and how it will be used. Some doctors fear a punitive approach will be adopted for those who fail to conform for whatever reason, while others question whether it will actually improve patient care or if it is simply another bureaucratic box-ticking exercise.

While appraisal has provided a basis for determining education and development plans it will now contribute to the revalidation process, with your revalidation folder containing information on how well you are practising with evidence of your continuing professional development. Annual appraisals will be the principal method for you to demonstrate you are meeting the standards required for revalidation. However, the GMC has acknowledged that the quality of appraisals differs in various parts of the UK and may not always be adequate for revalidation purposes.

Professional development portfolios specific to all specialties are now provided by the medical royal colleges and maintained by all doctors and provide some of the evidence on which appraisal is based. Concerns about a doctor's fitness to practise should have been raised long before appraisal. There should be no surprises at the revalidation stage.

Thus, appraisal for revalidation is essentially similar to trainee appraisal and the GMC has developed a framework for appraisal and assessment that aims to support the delivery of revalidation. For this the GMC reviewed *Good Medical Practice* and derived from it attributes that cover the core requirements of good practice. This was elaborated into a framework, which shows suggested generic standards and possible sources of evidence. The attributes are categorised into four domains (outlined below).

The details of the framework for appraisal and assessment are available at the GMC website (www.gmc-uk.org/doctors/licensing/docs/Framework_4_3.pdf). Divided into four domains, it defines the attributes, generic standards and possible sources of evidence. The main headings are as follows.

o Knowledge, Skills and Performance:
  ‣ maintaining professional performance
  ‣ applying knowledge and experience to practice
  ‣ clear, accurate and legible records.
o Safety and Quality:
  ‣ putting into effect systems to protect patients and improve care
  ‣ respond to risks to safety
  ‣ protect patients and colleagues from any risk posed by your health.
o Communication, Partnership and Teamwork:
  ‣ communicate effectively
  ‣ work constructively with colleagues and delegate effectively
  ‣ establish and maintain partnerships with patients.
o Maintaining Trust
  ‣ show respect for patients
  ‣ treat patients and colleagues fairly and without discrimination
  ‣ act with honesty and integrity.

Because this is about to be introduced at the time of writing you are advised to visit www.gmc-uk.org/doctors/licensing/index.asp for up-to-date information, and the link to Revalidation FAQs may be useful in answering your queries and concerns.

360-degree feedback

One element required by the GMC for revalidation is participation in an independent process for obtaining feedback from patients (if applicable) and colleagues, also known as multisource feedback (MSF) or 360-degree feedback.

One feedback is required in the first two years and one in the final two years of the five-year revalidation cycle. Reflections and changes need to be demonstrated and the second MSF should show improvement in areas of concern highlighted by the first MSF or reflection on why no improvement has been observed.

The GMC has been developing patient and colleague questionnaires for use within the revalidation process based on the standards contained in *Good Medical Practice*. Early research by Peninsula Medical School into the validity, reliability and practicality of the questionnaires has been encouraging.

There have also been more extensive pilot studies to test the psychometric performance of the questionnaires and look further into their feasibility and the operational rules for their possible use. This independent research has found that questionnaires have the potential to be a reliable means of collecting information regarding doctors' performance.

The results of the pilot study conducted by Professor John Campbell of Peninsula Medical School were published in June 2008. The full article is online in the *Quality and Safety in Health Care Journal* (available at qshc.bmj.com/cgi/content/full/17/3/18 7?ijkey=MoqPsZPEEq2w2&keytype=ref&siteid=bmjjournals).

The draft GMC colleague and patient questionnaires are also available to read at the GMC and Doctors.net website, although it is noted they may be subject to changes depending on the outcomes of the further research.

The most often heard complaint about the 360-degree feedback is: 'How can a secretary judge me?' Well, the secretary is not there to judge or to give feedback on medical competence but to give feedback on other competences such as communicating, administrative functioning, and the like.

The validity and reliability of the approach was demonstrated in a study undertaken in Canada (Hall *et al.* 1999) and other studies have generally shown that 360-degree feedback improved the performance of consultants receiving the feedback. A more recent study in the UK (Campbell *et al.* 2008) concluded that

> GMC patient and colleague questionnaires offered a reliable basis for the assessment of professionalism among UK doctors. If used in the revalidation of doctors' registration they would be capable of discriminating a range of professional performance among doctors and potentially identifying a minority whose practice should be subjected to further scrutiny.

Lelliott *et al.* (2008) found that reliable 360-degree assessment of humane judgement is feasible for psychiatrists who work in large multi-professional teams and who have large caseloads. However, for balance, a paper (Overeem *et al.* 2009) showed that out of 23 consultants only 11 made concrete steps towards performance improvement.

But which factors promote or block implementation of the suggestions received by consultants during a 360-degree feedback?

Overall, 360-degree feedback can work if skilled facilitators are available to encourage reflection, concrete goals are set and follow-up interviews are planned. The main obstruction to the good use of 360-degree feedback is an existing lack of openness in hospitals, departments or consultant groups. The other important factor is absence of constructive feedback.

This is an opportunity to briefly mention the subject of giving good feedback, although advice is given in more detail in Chapter 3.

o Be clear about what you want to say.
o Start by emphasizing the positive.
o Be specific. Avoid general comments and clarify pronouns such as 'it', 'that', etc.
o Focus on behaviour that you have seen or observed rather than the person.
o Refer to behaviour that can be changed.
o Be descriptive rather than evaluative. Avoid qualifications.
o Own the feedback. Use 'I' statements.
o Avoid generalisations and be specific with observed examples.
o If possible, let the appraisee work out for themselves how to improve performance.

Supporting and advising others
Mentoring

In Homer's *Odyssey*, as Odysseus is about to embark upon the Trojan wars he asks his friend Alimus whether his son Mentor might act as role model and advisor to his own son Telemachus while he is away.

What is mentoring?

There are now many definitions of mentoring. The dictionary defines 'mentor' as 'experienced and trusted advisor' (*Oxford*) and 'wise or trusted advisor or guide' (*Collins*), although The Standing Committee on Postgraduate Medical and Dental Education (SCOPME) defined it as

> The process whereby an experienced, highly regarded, empathic person (the mentor), guides another individual (the mentee) in the development and re-examination of their own ideas, learning, and personal and professional development. The mentor, who often but not necessarily works in the same organisation or field as the mentee, achieves this by listening and talking in confidence to the mentee. (SCOPME 1996)

Some colleges, such as the Royal College of Surgeons England, use this definition throughout all guidance and recommendations on mentoring.

Other research defines mentoring based on what it is not; for example, Connor and Pokora (2007) contrast mentoring with patronage and therapy. The London Deanery, which has carried out some work on mentoring in the medical environment (*see* below), explains the differences. Others define mentoring by comparing it with counselling, coaching and job planning and again the work of the London Deanery demonstrates the differences. Also various models of mentoring exist and according to Arkutu and Rock (2006) the two most often cited in the medical context are 'Egan Skilled Helper' and the '5 C Model'. The work by the London Deanery is available at www.mentoring.londondeanery.ac.uk/mentees/introduction and is a very useful source of material on the subject. It includes an introduction to the process – what a mentor does, what makes mentoring work, the skills needed, ground rules, agreements and contracts, ethical codes of practice, recording sheets, developing reflective practice and evaluation forms.

Mentoring has become increasingly prominent in the NHS, after first appearing in management literature in the 1970s. Most of the colleges now strongly advocate mentoring at all stages of a trainee's education and throughout their career. The BMA lobbied for the development of mentoring schemes for all doctors. Most colleges now have publications, such as the RCS *Good Surgical Practice*, and are looking at ways of developing a culture of mentoring.

Why do doctors need mentoring?

The colleges agree that mentoring can be beneficial for doctors at any stage of their career and fully support participation in mentoring arrangements. There is certainly increasing interest in mentoring within the medical profession and it is promoted as an essential component of Modernising Medical Careers. Many trusts have set up mentoring schemes for other healthcare professionals and such schemes are being extended to include all clinical staff.

The RCS suggests that it should not just be associated with 'crisis points' in a surgeon's career, as mentoring targeted at specific groups, or at a specific milestone in a surgeon's career, may be beneficial. Examples of such points include the following.

○ Training within shorter hours under EWTD and within a streamlined training programme under MMC being stressful.
○ Newly appointed consultants finding the transition to first consultant appointment challenging.
○ Existing consultants having to work within an increasingly target-driven environment while providing training and support to less experienced surgeons.
○ Surgeons from diverse backgrounds may also face particular pressures and require support.

All these groups may require additional support and may benefit from a mentoring arrangement.

Skills for mentors and mentees

Some skills are required for both mentee and mentor. It can be perceived as an additional burden so training for participants in a mentoring relationship is important. According to London Deanery (2008) research, 'without training', only 3 out of 10 mentoring relationships have a positive result. With training that can be doubled; if you train both the mentor and the mentee you can get a success rate up to 9 out of 10 (Snell 1999).

For the mentor the following is a list of desirable attributes.

Good mentors should aim to:
○ listen and respond appropriately
○ share relevant personal experiences
○ form and nurture a mutual learning friendship
○ encourage the development of insight
○ act as a sounding board for ideas and problems
○ have clear goals
○ be good humoured
○ communicate well with peers and junior staff
○ have commitment to own learning.

Good mentors sometimes:
○ use coaching behaviours
○ use counselling behaviours
○ avoid undue criticism
○ challenge assumptions

o   act as a role model
o   open doors as sponsors.

Good mentors never:
o   discipline (there are other mechanisms for this)
o   condemn
o   appraise formally
o   assess for a third party
o   supervise.

When you are given a mentor how will you know if they are right for you? You will usually know in the first meeting whether you 'click' or not. If you do not feel comfortable at the end of a first meeting, you ought to be offered another mentor.

The benefits of mentoring

The benefits of mentoring have been widely documented and can include benefits for mentees, mentors and the organisation:
o   improve motivation
o   increase job satisfaction (useful with long-serving staff)
o   improve career progression
o   develop knowledge and skills
o   develop leadership skills
o   organisational level benefits such as:
  ›   improved commitment
  ›   supporting innovation
  ›   improved 'productivity'
  ›   better functioning teams
  ›   developing positive attitudes to change
  ›   reduced complaints
  ›   improved management of conflict (colleagues and patients)
  ›   improved retention of staff
  ›   improved succession planning.

Counselling

The British Association for Counselling and Psychotherapy (BACP) definition of counselling is where a client is seen in a private and confidential setting in order to explore a problem they may be experiencing. It can be difficult, however, to make a distinction between counselling and psychotherapy. There are well-founded traditions which use the terms interchangeably. A psychotherapist working in a hospital is likely to be concerned with severe psychological disorders. Counsellors working for voluntary agencies or in educational settings usually concentrate on 'everyday' problems and difficulties. Many are qualified to offer therapeutic work that in any other context would be called psychotherapy. It is worth remembering that counselling is always at the request of the client. No one can be 'sent' for counselling.

Personal counselling

Counselling requires specific training and should be conducted by an accredited counsellor. Professional counsellors should always be adequately supervised. Counsellors will always refer appropriately where necessary. Doctors are most likely to be involved where work-related performance is compromised. Counselling should not be confused with meddling, however well intentioned. It should always be non-judgemental, except when the law is broken.

Basic counselling skills can be useful and are available to doctors who wish to acquire additional competency. It will not make you an accredited and fully trained counsellor (this takes at least three years' training). Check your local Postgraduate Medical Centre (PGMC) or go online for current availability.

Before enrolling on a course it is advisable to be aware of its theoretical emphasis and what that means in terms of the learning experience offered and the skills acquired. There are different methods of counselling. Most courses start from a theoretical base – typically humanistic, psychodynamic, cognitive or behavioural.

Sometimes doctors may be required to help or advise colleagues, regardless of whether they have any knowledge of, or ability to provide, counselling. By default or design it can be assumed doctors are naturally well placed to offer solace and wisdom. Some problems will be beyond the expertise of many, even the most empathic, and an understanding of one's own limitations can be crucial. Offering advice on how to obtain suitable information will be a more appropriate option.

Counselling skills should ideally include:
- acknowledging a problem exists
- enabling change to reduce confusion/anxiety
- encouraging and developing insight
- acceptance and understanding of others.

It will not include:
- solving all problems
- removing all distress
- saying what you would do
- being judgemental.

Appropriate action may include:
- listening
- encouraging
- exploring options.

The most valuable skill is the ability to listen. (For more information on effective listening *see* Chapter 3.) Problems can often be alleviated or minimised by the simple expedient of having someone prepared to listen. Listening should never be underestimated.

Career counselling

Do you loathe Monday mornings, live for holidays, wonder why you became a doctor, dread yet another clinic? SCOPME considered that career counselling should be a part of appraisal (Clayton 1998) because appraisal is a tool to help career development and it is often in that situation that the subject surfaces.

There are two issues here, depending on whether you are seeking counselling or being drawn into a situation where someone else needs it. In either situation some knowledge of what is available might help you or help you to direct someone in the right direction.

Occasionally, doctors have physical, emotional or psychological problems that might have an impact on their future career choice. If you need confidential help or support, you can refer yourself or your trainee to your trust's occupational health service or access other support services through your postgraduate deanery.

Undertaking career counselling uses methods to assess attitudes, values, personal attributes, skills and knowledge to help make career choices. This may be necessary for doctors (and medical students) who are at or before a crossroads in their careers. Career counselling requires the counsellor to have counselling skills, a wide range of knowledge of medical careers and ready access to career information and the consequences of each choice.

For many appraisers this is simply not possible, so the appraiser may be only the conduit to pass the trainee on to someone appropriate. There is a danger of career counselling developing into career advice and persuasion followed by patronage, leading to unfairness and a potentially poor career choice.

Career counselling seems to have become a burgeoning industry and there are a number of websites offering advice and counselling sessions for up to £500 per session! Anita Houghton (2005) has written a useful book for those interested in reflecting on their personal career preferences.

Career guidance

Career guidance differs from career counselling in that the individual is advised or is providing advice about an already chosen career pathway. Guidance usually requires someone to have a detailed knowledge of that particular career pathway and may include assessment of the stage of training reached. Career counselling and career guidance are sometimes confused and used interchangeably. It is important that it is clear whether the process is about making a career choice between a variety of careers or dealing with an already chosen career. MMC has led to the introduction of more structured approaches to early career advice.

For trainees, some deaneries are evaluating career planning tools like Sci59 or Myers-Briggs (*see* Chapter 1) which help you understand yourself better and can point you in the direction of a career that might suit you. These tools seldom provide the 'answer' to planning a career in medicine but may be a useful place to start a discussion with peers, supervisor or career advisor.

Here are a few websites that could help you down the path of decisiveness. I have no personal experience of any of them and their inclusion does not imply any recommendation. I add them all only because they have been drawn to my attention as sources of information. Some provide overlap service between career advice and emotional support (*see* below under health issues).

- **BMJ Careers** in addition to being a place to look for your next job will enable you to find a huge range of career-related articles covering everything from policy to working in a particular specialty, with tips on how to construct a winning CV. It also provides information about career opportunities in medicine and related fields. In the Careers Advice Zone there is an interactive and impartial careers advice service. Go to www.bmjcareers.com.
- **NHS Medical Careers** will support medical students and doctors in training as they plan their specialty careers. It is designed to provide a structured, organised method of choosing a specialty and uses a four-stage approach to career planning. It combines interactive tools and some of the most in-depth information around all specialties in one place. Go to www.medicalcareers.nhs.uk. There are also links to it at www.nhsemployers.org and www.foundationprogramme.nhs.uk.
- **Local Deanery** sites describe the specialty training opportunities available together with contact details for training programmes. Go to www.foundationprogramme. nhs.uk/deaneries for a full list of deaneries in the UK and links to their websites.
- **MedNet** provides doctors and dentists working in the area covered by the London Deanery with practical advice about their career, emotional support should they need it and, if appropriate, access to brief or longer term psychotherapy. The service operates on a strictly confidential basis. For counselling and support, Tel: 020 8938 2411, or go to www.londondeanery.ac.uk/var/MedNet.
- **Medical royal colleges** are responsible for setting the standards for specialty training and provide information about current and future specialty training pathways, requirements and curricula.
- **UK Foundation Programme Office** provides information for medical students, foundation doctors and those involved in delivering the Foundation Programme across the UK. Go to www.foundationprogramme.nhs.uk.
- **Healthcare Performance** works with individual doctors and/or their employers on a number of issues that can affect performance and careers. They provide one-to-one coaching and support for doctors as well as career coaching, and also work with groups of doctors to help improve their team skills and interpersonal and professional behaviours. Tel: 01892 724245. Email: info@healthcareperformance. co.uk www.healthcareperformance.co.uk.
- **Medical Forum** provides a career guidance programme for those who are thinking about a change in career direction. Tel: 07000 7901 7318. www.medicalforum.com.
- **Medical Women's Federation** represents the interests of women doctors to government and national bodies, bringing together women trying to advance their medical careers. Tel: 020 7387 7765. Email: admin.mwf@btconnect.com or go to www.medicalwomensfederation.org.uk.
- **Women in Surgical Training – The Royal College of Surgeons of England** have a mission to encourage, enable and inspire women to fulfil their surgical ambitions. Tel: 020 7869 6212. Email: wist@rcseng.ac.uk, or go to www.rcseng.ac.uk.

Poorly performing colleagues

Just as with anyone else, situations can occur in a doctor's life that affect their work. It could be personal problems involving family members, a breakdown of a relationship or health problems. With appraisal, assessment, recertification and revalidation these problems are more likely to surface at an early stage. Generally, they are likely to fall into one of four areas:

o   personal conduct
o   professional conduct
o   competence and performance issues
o   health and sickness issues.

Early detection is the most crucial factor because experience has shown that early intervention is often best. Indeed the GMC (2006) stress that it is your duty to

> protect patients from risk of harm posed by another colleague's conduct, performance or health. The safety of patients must come first at all times. If you have concerns that a colleague may not be fit to practise you must take appropriate steps without delay. Concerns must be investigated and patients protected where necessary. This means you must give an honest explanation of your concerns to an appropriate person from your employing or contracting body and follow their procedures.

Many problems can be resolved at a local level, rather than involving all the formal processes. However, the principles of finding out and using facts, and not opinions, will hopefully work well in most cases.

The role of the employer

Trusts and employers will have procedures laid down for discipline, performance and sickness issues. Human resources will be able to provide advice regarding the trust's procedural and legal matters. But do check your facts before taking action, making sure issues are not based merely on opinions.

Personal conduct issues

Personal conduct issues include such things as theft, fraud, assault on another member of staff, vandalism, rudeness, bullying, racial and sexual harassment, downloading pornography from a computer in the library and attitude problems in relation to colleagues, other staff and patients. The trust (as the employer) will take the lead under its approved disciplinary procedures.

Professional conduct issues

Problems include research misconduct, failure to take consent properly, prescribing issues, improper relationships with patients, improper certification issues (such as the signing of cremation forms, sickness certification and passport forms) as well as breach of confidentiality. In the case of trainees the employing trust will take the lead under its disciplinary procedures and also inform the deanery in writing at the earliest stage.

The deanery will provide an input into such a disciplinary process and will involve the clinical supervisor, educational supervisor, possibly the clinical tutor, specialty college tutor or other member of the deanery, depending on local arrangements and the seniority of the doctors within the training programme. Any decision to involve the GMC is a serious one for the doctor involved and this will be a joint decision between the trust (or other employer) and the deanery.

Competence and performance issues

These issues may involve a single serious mistake or poor clinical outcomes (perhaps found as a result of audit), poor timekeeping, poor communication skills, poor consultation skills and repeated failure to attend educational events. Local disciplinary procedures will be followed or, for trainees, this type of problem may be dealt with through the educational framework. The Educational Supervisor and Clinical Supervisor will take a lead in some of these problems. Postgraduate deaneries may also provide further expert assessment and remedial training in such areas of communication and consultation skills.

An isolated serious mistake could happen to anyone. Many doctors have been in this situation at some time in their careers. It does not necessarily reflect the overall competence of the doctor concerned (NPSA 2005). Complexity brings risks and evidence shows that things will and do go wrong and that patients are sometimes harmed no matter how dedicated and professional the staff.

The National Patient Safety Agency (NPSA) lists 'Seven Steps' that are core to patient safety. Each guide in the series (there's one for each of primary care, general practice, mental health and a full reference guide) provides a checklist to help staff to plan their activities and measure patient safety performance. This helps to ensure that the care provided is as safe as possible, and that when things do go wrong the right action is taken. They will also help healthcare organisations to meet clinical governance, risk management and control assurance targets. You can find them at www.nrls.npsa.nhs.uk/resources/collections/seven-steps-to-patient-safety/.

Such a mistake might lead to a formal inquiry. For trainees it is important that the local deanery be kept informed. Counselling and pastoral support should be available as such an event can be highly stressful for all concerned. In the past doctors in this situation were often suspended. The Chief Medical Officer has asked trusts to try to avoid suspending doctors in such circumstances. Instead they should consider the possibility of a referral to the National Clinical Assessment Service (NCAS).

If the doctor's performance is consistently poor even though all educational measures have been tried to put things right, it may be necessary to inform the GMC. This is not a decision to be taken lightly or on the spur of the moment. Such a referral may have momentous and unpredictable consequences for the doctor concerned. In the case of a trainee this will again need to be a joint decision between the trust and the deanery.

Involving the GMC

If there are no appropriate local systems, or the local systems do not resolve the problem, and you are still concerned about the safety of patients you should inform the relevant regulatory body. If you are not sure what to do, discuss your concerns with an impartial colleague or contact your defence body, a professional organisation or the GMC for advice.

If you have management responsibilities, make sure that systems are in place through which colleagues can raise concerns about risks to patients, and you must follow the GMC guidance in *Management for Doctors*.

The GMC in 2009 produced a number of useful sources on poorly performing doctors and these can all be accessed from their main website. This is particularly useful to be aware of should you ever have to be involved in taking action to protect patients. In 2009 the GMC noted a huge rise in the number of doctors being reported to it with concerns over their fitness to practise (up 30% on 2008). This may suggest that trusts are clamping down on poorly performing doctors in advance of revalidation.

The amount of material and advice is beyond the scope of this section but, briefly, the GMC may take action if a doctor's fitness to practise is impaired for the following reasons:

o misconduct
o deficient performance
o a criminal conviction or caution in the British Isles (or elsewhere for an offence which would be a criminal offence if committed in England or Wales)
o physical or mental ill-health
o a decision by a regulatory body either in the British Isles or overseas.

Where a doctor's fitness to practise is found to be impaired, it can suspend or remove a doctor from the medical register or place conditions on the doctor's registration. They can also issue a warning to a doctor where the doctor's fitness to practise is not impaired but there has been a significant departure from the principles set out in the GMC's guidance for doctors, *Good Medical Practice*.

The GMC's procedures are divided into two separate stages:

o investigate the case to assess whether to refer it for adjudication
o adjudication by a 'Fitness to Practice' panel.

An 'Interim Orders Panel' can also suspend or place conditions on a doctor's registration while the GMC's investigation continues.

For further information a pamphlet called *A Guide for Doctors Referred to the GMC* can be downloaded at www.gmc-uk.org/concerns/doctors_under_investigation/a_guide_for_referred_doctors.asp.

Health issues

Studies have shown that doctors exhibit a relatively high level of mental health problems, particularly depression, which may lead to drug abuse and suicide (Tyssen and Vaglum 2002). Symptoms, particularly of depression, were highest during the first postgraduate year. Factors such as family background, personality traits (neuroticism and self-criticism) and coping by wishful thinking as well as contextual factors including perceived medical-school stress, perceived overwork, emotional pressure, working in an intensive-care setting and stress outside work were often predictive of mental health problems.

The *Australian Manual of Mental Health Care in General Practice* states that around 20% of medical students exhibit obsessive-compulsive personality traits, including perfectionism, isolation of affect, conscientiousness and a need to feel 'in control'. These traits are in many respects adaptive to the demands of the job. However, they also place the doctor at risk. Perfectionism may contribute to a high level of performance but at the expense of high levels of anxiety and excessive self-criticism if something goes wrong. It is an asset to be a good organiser but this trait can lead to personality clashes with others who also like to be in control. Obsessive-compulsive traits may place the individual at risk of depression and anxiety.

Traits characteristic of the Type A personality are also common among doctors – competitiveness, feelings of time pressure, impatience and irritability. Traits that are adaptive in many situations, they are also associated with increased physical and psychological morbidity.

Clinical work is often very stressful. Doctors are exposed to the whole gamut of human suffering, including death and dying. They may hear stories of abuse and even torture. Some of their patients will be difficult and demanding. Treating colleagues and their families is often identified as being particularly stressful. Doctors often need to make difficult ethical judgements, balancing conflicting demands for example between the need to maintain confidentiality versus the requirement to report abuse. They are often powerless to cure and limited in their ability to minimise suffering limitations that patients and their families are not always immediately willing to acknowledge. Doctors are constrained by standards of behaviour that are more exacting than those applied in most other professions. In addition, female doctors face role strain, having to strike a balance between the demands of work and family.

Doctors have distinct vulnerabilities to drug and alcohol addiction (Fozard 2009). There is a tendency to present late due to shame, guilt, fear of breach of confidentiality and fear of GMC procedures and many doctors do not seek help through conventional avenues but rather through the 'old boy's network'. Additionally, there is a reticence among colleagues to intervene despite a doctor's duty to protect the health of both patients and colleagues. If done early enough, involvement with the GMC can facilitate a good outcome and a doctor can return to work in recovery. Left late, outcomes may not be as good.

It is often said that doctors aren't always very good patients and this is never truer than when they may be suffering from a problem with drink or drugs. Medical students are often described as drinking to excess but the path from a 'boozy night' to a lecture hall doesn't seem hard to cope with when there is no patient to deal with. When facing night-shifts, a mortgage, children and maybe a couple of divorces it suddenly becomes very different.

Yet a professional veneer can hide a vulnerable human being desperate for help. There have been very public exposés of prominent doctors with drink and drug problems over the last decade. Maybe with earlier intervention by colleagues and improved help these public personality assassinations can be avoided. As a victim once put it, 'Don't let a crisis become a catastrophe.'

The *Good Medical Practice* (GMC 2009) stresses that doctors are under a professional duty to take steps to protect patients from a risk of harm posed by other health professionals. If you believe a colleague's performance or health is a threat to patient safety, the GMC also has *A Guide for Health Professionals on How to Report a Doctor to the GMC* (GMC 2009). You must protect patients from risk of harm posed by another colleague's conduct, performance or health. If you have concerns that a colleague may not be fit to practise, you must take appropriate steps without delay so that the concerns are investigated and patients protected where necessary. This means you must give an honest explanation of your concerns to an appropriate person from your employing or contracting body, and follow their procedures.

Most doctors who are ill never need come to the GMC's attention. Where there are good local systems to support and supervise sick doctors there is normally no need to refer to the GMC provided that the sick doctor takes and follows independent advice about the nature and extent of professional practice.

If there are no appropriate local systems, or local systems do not resolve the problem, and you are still concerned about the safety of patients you should inform the relevant regulatory body. If you are not sure what to do, discuss your concerns with an impartial colleague or contact your defence body, a professional organisation or the GMC for advice.

Referral to the GMC is likely to be appropriate where the doctor's illness is impacting (or may impact) on his or her professional performance and, in addition, one or more of the following also applies:

o the doctor's ill health is posing, or may pose, a risk to patients
o the doctor refuses or has failed to follow advice and guidance from his or her own doctor, occupational health adviser or employer
o the doctor's conduct has led to the involvement of the police and/or the courts or raised other concerns.

If you have management responsibilities, make sure that systems are in place through which colleagues can raise concerns about risks to patients and you must follow the guidance in *Management for Doctors* (GMC 2006).

Before taking any action it is important to ascertain the facts and it is often helpful and certainly sensible to discuss your concerns with an experienced senior colleague before notifying the employing authority or regulatory body.

The guide also stresses that you should be registered with a general practitioner outside your family to ensure that you have access to independent and objective medical care and should not treat yourself.

You should protect your patients, your colleagues and yourself by being immunised against common serious communicable diseases where vaccines are available.

If you know that you have, or think that you might have, a serious condition that you could pass on to patients, or if your judgement or performance could be affected by a condition or its treatment, you must consult a suitably qualified colleague. You must ask for and follow their advice about investigations, treatment and changes to your practice that they consider necessary. You must not rely on your own assessment of the risk you pose to patients.

Prevention is better than cure

Regular and constructive day-to-day feedback is one of the best ways to help trainees learn. Regular appraisal and assessments are essential and can do a great deal to identify and help address performance problems before they become serious.

Record maintenance is an important aspect of supervision. Notes should be kept of meetings held to discuss the doctor's adherence to agreed and accepted processes such as the use of guidelines, furthering their own education, attendance at protected teaching sessions, contribution to research and development activities, audit, and their awareness of their own clinical outcomes. In the absence of written evidence of meetings the poorly performing doctor may then often claim that they were completely unaware of any problem. Appraisals and assessments must be documented. Keep copies of all assessments and appraisals. Always make notes of performance-related meetings, conversations and so on and keep copies.

The GMC guidance *Good Medical Practice* (GMC 2006) stresses your duty to protect patients if you believe a colleague's performance or health is a threat. This was discussed earlier in this chapter under 'Health issues'.

The Central Consultants and Specialists Committee (CCSC) has also produced guidance on the actions that consultants should take if they are concerned about the performance of colleagues. They highlight the following.

○ Act quickly to protect patients.
○ Place clear professional responsibility and take action where there are serious concerns.
○ The first step may be to discuss the problem with a senior colleague or a colleague in a specialty from another hospital.
○ Consider the use of local informal procedures.
○ Possibly seek advice from the local BMA office.
○ It may be necessary to bring the matter to the attention of your trust through the Medical Director, Clinical Director or even the Chief Executive.

There are a number of agencies available to help doctors in these situations.

There are services for doctors with drug or alcohol problems, although not yet nationwide. Any medical student or doctor who wants advice or support can currently access it at www.support4doctors.org. This website also provides links to resources such as the Doctors' and Dentists' Group, a group that helps doctors and dentists in recovery from substance abuse. Another potentially useful service featured is the Doctors Support Network, a confidential service for doctors who have mental health problems.

The 2007 white paper *Trust, Assurance and Safety: the regulation of health professionals in the 21st century* proposed a pilot service for doctors with health problems and a national advisory group. The DoH agreed three years' funding for a prototype service that would provide care with additional safeguards to ensure confidentiality and privacy, and ensuring doctors treating doctors have an appropriate level of expertise.

The National Clinical Assessment Service was given the task of designing and commissioning a prototype Practitioner Health Programme (PHP) on behalf of the Department of Health. The product of this is a primary care-led service based at the Hurley Group's Riverside Medical Centre in Vauxhall, London. It is a free, confidential service for doctors and dentists who have mental or physical health concerns and/or addiction problems and who live or work in the London area.

A doctor with specialist mental health and addiction expertise has drawn together a multidisciplinary team which includes an occupational therapist, a nurse specialising in addictions and a psychologist. The team works closely with secondary care experts from the South London and Maudsley Foundation Trust, Tavistock and Portman Foundation Trust and Capio Nightingale. The benefits are huge; patients can see both primary and secondary care experts at Riverside, and can be referred to a myriad of inpatient, outpatient and therapy services. The aim is to provide a fast and responsive service. Patients are guaranteed an appointment within 48 hours but may be seen on the same day if necessary. The joint primary and secondary care team meet weekly to discuss individual patients' progress. Because the service is specific to the needs of doctors the complexity of the doctor–patient relationship and confidentiality are key parts of the service.

Sick doctors also have access to the following contacts.

○ **Association of Anaesthetists' Sick Doctor Scheme:** Advice for anaesthetists. Tel: 020 7631 1650.
○ **Association of Anaesthetists Sick Doctor Scheme of Great Britain and Ireland:** Tel: 0171 631 1650 (0900 – 1730).
○ **Association of Medical Professionals with Hearing Loss:** AMPHL provides information, promotes advocacy and mentorship, and creates a network for individuals with hearing loss interested in or working in healthcare fields. Go to www. amphl.org
○ **BMA's Doctors with Disabilities**
○ **BMA Counselling Service:** Provides 24/7 telephone counselling by qualified counsellors. Tel: 08459 200 169, or go to www.bma.org.uk.
○ **BMA Doctors for Doctors Service:** Provides help for doctors in employment difficulties, especially in relation to mental health problems and abuse of alcohol and drugs. The unit provides a signposting service to the area of help that is most pertinent to the individual doctor's needs. Tel: 020 7383 6739.
○ **British Doctors' and Dentists' Group:** A network of support groups for recovering medical and dental drug and alcohol users. Students are also welcomed. The groups are accessed via the Medical Council on Alcohol. Tel: 020 7487 4445, or go to www.m-c-a.org.uk.
○ **British International Doctors' Association:** Where cultural or linguistic problems may be a contributing factor doctors can access the health counselling panel. Tel: 0161 456 7828. Email: bida@btconnect.com.
○ **Clinicians' Health Intervention Treatment and Support:** Promotes a consistent response to the problem of substance misuse among clinical staff throughout the

UK. Tel: 01335 342144. Email: avoca@birdsgrove.freeserve.co.uk.

o **Deaf Professionals Network:** This group provides an opportunity to network and share experiences. The website is primarily for deaf professionals who live in and around London. This website can also be used as a resource for other deaf professionals who cannot attend the network meetings. www.deafprofessionals.com Email: enquiries@deafprofessionals.com.

o **Doctors' Support Network and Doctors' Support Line:** Self-help organisations for doctors with work difficulties, anxiety, depression, or family problems.

o **Doctors' Support Network:** Tel: 0871 245 8376, or go to www.dsn.org.uk Email: secretary@dsn.org.uk.

o **Doctors' Support Line:** Tel: 0870 765 0001, or go to www.doctorssupportline.org Email: info@dsn.org.uk.

o **Hope 4 Medics:** A support group for doctors with disabilities. Go to www.hope4 medics.co.uk/about.php Email: info@hope4medics.co.uk.

o **NHS Practitioner Health Programme:** A free confidential service for doctors and dentists who have mental or physical health concerns and/or addiction problems in particular where this may be affecting their work. Go to www.php.nhs.uk.

o **Primary Care Support Service:** Provided for GPs, dentists and community pharmacists in Wales, run as an independent service and funded by the Welsh Assembly. The facility offers counselling, support, education and information. Tel: 01248 388288, or go to www.wales.nhs.uk.

o **Psychiatrists' Support Service – Royal College of Psychiatrists:** A confidential support and advice telephone helpline to assist doctors in difficulty. Doctors who contact the service must be Members or Associates of the College who may be experiencing difficulties over the following: addictions, bullying and harassment, career pathway, discrimination, examinations, involvement with the General Medical Council or the National Clinical Assessment Service – this is not an exhaustive list. Tel: 0207 245 0412 for the Psychiatrists' Support Service manager. Email: psychiatristssupportservice@rcpsych.ac.uk.

o **Royal College of Obstetricians and Gynaecologists:** Provides mentoring support for Fellows and Members in difficulties. Tel: +44 (0)20 7772 6369. Email: cdhillon@rcog.org.uk.

o **Royal College of Surgeons Confidential Support and Advice Services for Surgeons (CSAS):** Offers a confidential telephone line as a point of personal contact between surgeons which is intended to offer a listening ear and will act as an informed signpost to appropriate sources of advice and support. Tel: 020 7869 6030, or go to www.rcseng.ac.uk Email: csas@rcseng.ac.uk.

o **Royal Medical Benevolent Fund:** Provides financial help for sick doctors. Tel: 020 8540 9194, or go to www.support4doctors.org.

o **Sick Doctors' Trust:** A pro-active service and self-help organisation for addicted physicians. Provides early intervention and treatment for addiction to alcohol or drugs. Tel: 0870 444 5163, or go to www.sick-doctors-trust.co.uk.

o **Take Time:** A wholly confidential service specifically for junior doctors and dentists in the Yorkshire Deanery who need help with work-related and personal difficulties which may cause anxiety, stress, depression and unhappiness. Tel: 0113 343 4642. Email: taketime@leeds.ac.uk.

Help may often be obtainable from the doctor's own GP, medical defence organisation, the NHS occupational health service, the postgraduate deanery and the LMC.

Details of the General Medical Council's role in helping sick doctors can be found at www.gmc-uk.org.

There are also doctor-specific sources for doctors or their bereaved spouses, partners and dependants with financial problems, as well as for doctors from minority ethnic groups and refugee and overseas qualified doctors. Online searches will access them but they are too numerous to mention here.

GMC's *Management for Doctors* (2006) is available to download at www.gmc-uk. org/guidance/current/library/management_for_doctors.asp.

Key learning points

- Preparation – teaching and appraisal are each made more effective if both trainer and trainee come prepared.
- Agenda – appraisal meetings should follow an agenda which should be agreed before or at the start of the meeting.
- Giving feedback – negative feedback is sometimes made more acceptable if it is preceded by positive remarks about the appraisee's performance. Even better, get them to tell you about the weaker areas of their performance.
- Setting objectives – all objectives should meet the criteria of being SMART.
- Dealing with conflict – if conflict is not easily resolved, the trainee should be transferred to the responsibility of another trainer.
- Manage confidentiality – as confidentiality can be crucial in getting the appraisee to be honest about weaknesses, it must be made clear that behaviour that contravenes GMC or other regulations will lead to disclosure to others.
- Avoid taking on a trainee's problems that may simply be about training activities. The trainee should carry some responsibility for organising his or her own learning. You should recognise that your role as an appraiser does not make you an expert counsellor. If serious problems are disclosed, refer them to someone who is better equipped to help them.

Related reading

Arkutu N, Rock WP. Does mentoring have a role in orthodontic training programmes? *Journal of Orthodontics*. 2006; **33**: 142–6.

Bilkhu J *et al. The Development of Quality Standards for GP Appraisal and Appraisers*. London: Royal College of General Practitioners; 2007.

British Medical Association (BMA). *Appraisal: a guide for medical practitioners*. London: British Medical Association; 2003.

British Medical Association (BMA). *Statement of Principles on Revalidation*. London:

British Medical Association; 2008. Available online at: www.bma.org.uk/images/BMA statementrevalidation_tcm41-173593.pdf

Bulstrode C, Hunt V. *Educating Consultants*. Oxford: Oxford University Press; 1996.

Campbell JL *et al*. Assessing the professional performance of UK doctors: an evaluation of the utility of the General Medical Council patient and colleague questionnaires. *Quality and Safety in Health Care*. 2008; **17**: 187–93.

Castle N, Garton H, Kenward G. Confidence vs. competence: basic life support skills of health professionals. *British Journal of Nursing*. 2007; **16**: 664–6.

Chief Medical Officer. *Trust, Assurance and Safety: the regulation of health professionals in the 21st century*. London: Department of Health; 2007.

Clayton B. Letter. *BMJ*. 1998; **316**: 75.

COGPED. *Deanery Role in Respect of GP Appraisal and Revalidation*. London: Committee of General Practice Education Directors; 2007.

Connor M, Pokora J. *Coaching and Mentoring at Work: developing effective practice*. Maidenhead: Open University Press; 2007.

Department of Health. *Appraisal for Doctors in Training in the NHS*. London: Department of Health; 2003.

Department of Health. *Good Doctors, Safer Patients*. London: Department of Health; 2006.

Foster-Turner J. *Coaching and Mentoring in Health and Social Care: the essential manual for professionals and organisations*. Oxford: Radcliffe Medical Press; 1995.

Fozard G. Drugs, drink and doctors: it could never happen to me . . . *Journal of Student Medical Sciences*. 18 July 2009.

Gatrell J, White T. *Medical Appraisal, Selection and Revalidation*. London: RSM Press; 2000.

General Medical Council (GMC). *The New Doctor*. London: GMC; 1997.

General Medical Council (GMC). *Licensing and Revalidation: formal guidance for doctors (draft)*. London: GMC; 2004.

General Medical Council (GMC). *Good Medical Practice: outlining set of core standards and values to which all doctors were expected to adhere in their everyday practice*. London: GMC; 2006, updated 2009. Available online with summary at: www.gmc-uk.org/static/documents/content/GMC_GMP_0911.pdf

General Medical Council (GMC). *Management for Doctors: guidance for doctors*. London: GMC; 2006. Available online at: www.gmc-uk.org/guidance/ethical_guidance/management_for_doctors.asp

General Medical Council (GMC). *A Guide for Health Professionals on How to Report a Doctor to the GMC*. London: GMC; 2009. Available online at: www.gmc-uk.org/FTP_proffesionals.pdf_snapshot.pdf

Gourlay R. *Dealing with Difficult Staff in the NHS*. London: Kogan Page; 1998.

Hall W *et al*. Assessment of physician performance in Alberta: the Physician Achievement Review. *Canadian Medical Association Journal*. 1999; **161**(1): 52–7.

Houghton A. *Know Yourself: the individual's guide to career development in healthcare*. Oxford: Radcliffe Medical Press; 2005.

Jelley D, Cheek B, Van Zwanenberg T. Quality assurance of general practitioner appraisal: successes and challenges in the Northern Deanery. *Education for Primary Care*. 2007; **18**: 180–91.

Kolb DA, Osland JS, Rubin IM. *Organizational Behaviour: an experiential approach*. 6th ed. Englewood Cliffs, New Jersey: Prentice-Hall; 2000.

Kurtz SM, Silverman J, Draper J. *Teaching and Learning Communication Skills in Medicine*. 2nd ed. Oxford: Radcliffe Publishing; 2005.

Lelliott P *et al.* Questionnaires for 360-degree assessment of consultant psychiatrists: development and psychometric properties. *The British Journal of Psychiatry.* 2008; **193**: 156–60.

Lewis M, Evans K. Quality assurance of GP appraisal: a two-year study. *Education for Primary Care;* 2006; **17**: 319–33.

Lewis M, Murray S, McKnight A, Chambers R. Revalidation: a role for postgraduate deaneries. *Education for Primary Care.* 2007; **18**(6): 674–83.

London Deanery. Mentoring. 2009. Available online at: www.mentoring.londondeanery. ac.uk/downloads/files/Mentoring%20overview%20current%20-%2020090601.pdf/? searchterm=Mentoring%20Overview

Marteau TM, Wynne G, Kaye W, Evans TR. Resuscitation: experience without feedback increases confidence but not skill. *BMJ.* 1990; **300**: 849–50.

MMC. *A Reference Guide for Postgraduate Specialty Training in the UK (the Gold Guide).* 3rd ed. London: Modernising Medical Careers; 2009.

NHS Clinical Governance Support Team (CGST). *Assuring the Quality of Medical Appraisal.* Leicester: CGST; 2006.

NHSE. *A Guide to Specialist Registrar Training (The Orange Book).* London: Department of Health; 1998.

NPSA. *Medical Error: how to avoid it all going wrong and what to do if it does.* London: National Patient Safety Organisation; 2005.

Overeem K, Wollersheim H, Driessen E *et al.* Doctors' perceptions of why 360-degree feedback does (not) work: a qualitative study. *Medical Education.* 2009; **43**(9): 874–82.

Pendleton D, Schofield T, Tate P. A method for giving feedback. In: Pendleton D, Schofield T, Tate P, Havelock P. *The Consultation: an approach to learning and teaching.* Oxford: Oxford University Press; 1984. pp. 68–71.

PMETB. *Workplace Based Assessment: a guide for implementation.* London: Postgraduate Medical Education and Training Board and Academy of Medical Royal Colleges; 2009. Available online at: www.pmetb.org.uk/fileadmin/user/QA/Assessment/PMETB_WPBA_ Guide_20090501.pdf

Ramsden P. *Learning to Teach in Higher Education.* 2nd ed. Abingdon: Routledge; 2003.

RCGP. *Portfolio of Evidence of Professional Standards for the Revalidation of General Practitioners.* London: Royal College of General Practitioners; 2004.

RCGP. *Good Medical Practice for GPs.* London: Royal College of General Practitioners; 2007.

RCGP. *The Principles of GP Appraisal.* London: Royal College of General Practitioners; 2008.

RCS. *Training the Trainers.* London; Raven Department of Education, The Royal College of Surgeons of England; 1996.

Rennie S. *Tossing Salads Too: a users' guide to medical student assessment.* Edinburgh: JASME; 2003.

Shaw K, MacKillop L, Armitage M. Revalidation, appraisal and clinical governance. *Clinical Governance: An International Journal.* 2007; **12**(3): 170–7.

Snell J. Head to head. *Health Service Journal.* 1999; **109**: 22–5.

Standing Committee on Postgraduate Medical and Dental Education (SCOPME). *Appraising Doctors and Dentists in Training: a working paper for consultation.* London: The Standing Committee on Postgraduate Medical and Dental Education; 1996.

Standing Committee on Postgraduate Medical and Dental Education (SCOPME). *Supporting Doctors and Dentists at Work: an enquiry into mentoring. A SCOPME Report.* The Standing Committee on Postgraduate Medical and Dental Education; 1998. Available online at: www. mcgl.dircon.co.uk/scopme/mentor5.pdf

Tyssen R, Vaglum P. Mental health problems among young doctors: an updated review of prospective studies. *Harvard Review of Psychiatry*. 2002; **10**(3): 154–65.

The UK Foundation Programme Office. *Rough Guide to Foundation Programme*. 2nd ed. London: TSO; 2007. Also available online at: www.foundationprogramme.nhs.uk

van der Vleuten C. The assessment of professional competence: developments, research and practical implications. *Advances in Health Sciences Education*. 1996; **1**: 41–67.

Effective interpersonal communication skills

This chapter provides a range of tools and techniques to help you in face-to-face communications in a wide range of settings. They include: effective listening, giving feedback, breaking bad news, core interviewing skills, presentation skills, contributing to meetings and being interviewed. Dealing with anger and complaints is covered in Chapter 4 (section on 'Dealing with anger') and Chapter 6 (section on 'Complaints').

Introduction: song, music and dance

We communicate with each other in order to give, seek and receive information; to inform, instruct, persuade, negotiate, motivate and encourage, to understand the opinions of others and so on. Interpersonal communication can be easy, happy and positive;

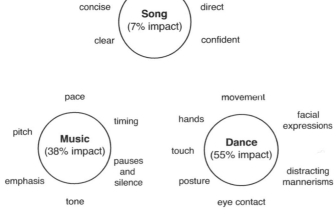

FIGURE 3.1 Song, music and dance

it can be difficult, uncomfortable and challenging, or it can be somewhere in between.

Various commentators are agreed that the impact on the listener in face-to-face communication is made up of 7% words, 38% voice tone and emphasis, and 55% body language. This is sometimes referred to as song, music and dance (*see* Figure 3.1).

Consider the anaesthetist who is reassuring a patient during the few minutes before they are taken into theatre. The effect of the doctor's hand on the patient's forearm as they hear the words has a far greater positive impact on their feelings than the words themselves.

This is not to suggest that the words that you use in, say, making a case for more resources, are not important – they may catch you out if you do not do your research. It is the longer-term impact on the experience of the listener that is enhanced by the other, non-verbal signals they receive.

The General Medical Council (GMC 2006) and other medical professional bodies including the Academy of Royal Medical Colleges, the Royal College of General Practitioners and the Royal College of Physicians all stress the importance of doctors developing good communication skills.

The GMC stress that to communicate effectively you must do the following.

○ Listen to patients, ask for and respect their views about their health and respond to their concerns and preferences.

○ Share information with patients in a way they can understand without being patronising. Provide the information they want or need to know about their condition, its likely progression and the treatment options available to them, including associated risks and uncertainties.

○ Respond to patients' questions and keep them informed about the progress of their care.

○ Make sure that patients are informed about how information is shared within teams and among those who will be providing their care.

○ Make sure, wherever practical, that arrangements are made to meet patients' language and communication needs.

Medical schools now provide communication skills training for medical students. The main subjects include breaking bad news, consulting patients and relatives, dealing with angry, difficult and reluctant patients, demonstrating empathy, and giving, explaining and receiving information. The skills are discussed mainly within this chapter, but like playing the piano or flying they cannot be mastered by reading how to do it, listening to a lecture or watching someone else do it. But this is often how doctors are expected to acquire their communication skills.

The GMC says there is an obligation on all doctors to review their skills as part of continuing professional development and take part in educational activities as a means of maintaining and further developing their competence (GMC 2006).

Doctors often face difficult situations, including bearing bad news, having to turn complex and often uncertain information into something that is understandable. They have to respond to the differing needs of a hugely diverse range of patients and their families, and do much of this when they are busy and under pressure. It is not surprising, therefore, that problems with communication can occur.

NHS Quality Improvement Scotland (Scottish Executive 2003) identified communication with patients as an issue that continues to give rise to concern. Indeed they state that it is one of the most common reasons for complaints from patients and is an important factor in litigation.

So when doctors use communication skills effectively there are a number of benefits (Maguire and Pitceathly 2002).

o Patients' problems are identified more accurately.
o Patients are more satisfied with their care and can better understand their problems.
o Patients are more likely to comply with treatment or lifestyle advice.
o Patients' distress and the vulnerability to anxiety and depression are lessened.
o The overall quality of care is improved by ensuring that patients' views are taken into account.
o Doctors' own well-being is improved.
o Fewer clinical errors are made.
o Patients are less likely to complain.
o There is a reduced likelihood of doctors being sued.

However, different patients require different approaches. Some patients may want only the minimal detail about their illness while others may challenge the information provided by doctors. There can be language barriers, learning difficulties and physical problems.

So what are the necessary communication skills and how can you acquire them? Communication looks easy when it is done well. But it requires engagement, empathy, an ability to listen and respond and it requires time.

The problems of communicating effectively have been acknowledged in reports produced by the British Medical Association (BMA 2004), identifying both personal and organisational barriers to effective communication.

The personal barriers

o Lack of skill and understanding – failure to understand the importance of using clear and simple language, giving structured explanations and listening to patients' views and encouraging two-way communication.
o Undervaluing the importance of communicating – for example, not appreciating the importance of keeping patients adequately informed.
o Negative attitudes by doctors towards communication and giving it a low priority due to their concern primarily to treat illness rather than focus on patients' other needs which may be psychological or related to social well-being.
o A lack of inclination to communicate – due to a lack of time, uncomfortable topics, lack of confidence and concerns relating to confidentiality.
o Human failings, such as tiredness and stress.
o Inconsistency of information. One of the biggest complaints from patients is of being given conflicting information by different healthcare professionals.
o Language difficulties – for some doctors who qualified in European countries who

are not required to take the English language test that is mandatory for other doctors from overseas.

The organisational barriers

Organisational barriers are usually outside a doctor's direct control and include:
○ lack of time
○ pressure of work
○ being subjected to interruptions.

The BMA report notes that doctors may be forced to devote less time to communicating with patients when the organisation they work for places an emphasis on increasing 'patient throughput' or similar initiatives.

Why it could be beneficial for you to enhance your communication skills

The Scottish Report referred to above stresses that there are also important benefits for doctors in improving job satisfaction and reducing the risk of burnout. The ability to intervene positively to improve people's lives should make medicine one of the most rewarding careers. Instead it is marked by high rates of suicide, emotional exhaustion, depersonalisation (treating people in an unfeeling, impersonal way) and a sense of low personal accomplishment. Ramirez and colleagues (2006) found evidence of stress-related psychiatric morbidity in 27% of consultants. They found that burnout was also more prevalent among consultants who felt insufficiently trained in communication and management skills.

There are other reasons (summarised above) why doctors need highly sophisticated interpersonal skills. Technical and clinical competence is essential but these qualities are insufficient to meet the challenges of this changing environment. Doctors also need support to help them respond effectively to these changing conditions.

Complaint handling

A poll commissioned by the Scottish Executive (2000) found that 23% of NHS users either have or have wanted to make a complaint about the service they received, although only 5% went on to raise an issue or make a complaint. This reflects a major culture change within society where many patients and their families are prepared to challenge the way services are provided.

Increasing litigation

Just as more people are willing to complain, more people are prepared to sue. In England the NHS expects to pay out £5 billion over the next few years. Poor handling of complaints contributes to increasing litigation. A survey carried out by Action Against Medical Accidents (AVMA) shows that most patients want an explanation of what went wrong and an apology but many are forced to take legal action when this is not forthcoming (ICM 2002).

Chronic disease management

More patients and their families are becoming 'experts' in their chronic conditions. The long-term management of conditions such as asthma, diabetes and epilepsy is also shifting to a partnership model – between patients and their doctors and between professionals in different disciplines. This is a profound change in the traditional role of the doctor and their relationship with patients and other professionals.

The appraisal process

The appraisal process demands a sophisticated level of communication skills if it is to be successful. Many consultants will be both appraisers and appraisees. Each role requires significant preparation and skills in the art of giving feedback. In addition, appraisal includes an 'assessment' of the appraisee's communication skills. This is therefore dealt with in more detail later in this chapter. The process of revalidation will require doctors to demonstrate effectiveness not only in what they do but how they do it, including how they interact and communicate with others.

Communication of risk

The awareness and quantification of risk is growing within the NHS and among the public. The delivery of healthcare is rarely risk free and trade-offs need be made between, for example, ease of access and safety. It is essential that clinicians are able to discuss risk with patients to help them make informed decisions.

Listening and giving feedback

Whether it is part of teaching, training, appraisal, mentoring, counselling or even taking a history, listening has to be effective. In addition in some situations you will need to give feedback, so it might be useful to consider these two skills in a little more detail.

Effective listening

Doctors, in common with others, are often in situations where they are supposed to be listening. It is easy to hear despite neither actively listening nor attending. Our minds can be distracted, a sign that can be noted by those on whom we should be concentrating. Effective (or active) listening is a developed skill and one worth acquiring. Effective listening obviously has many benefits, not least in a better understanding of what people say and feel. It can be hard work to acquire but can pay dividends. It will not come naturally to some people and may need practice to become proficient. There are a number of key elements to effective listening, as follows.

Concentrate

Try hard to concentrate on what is being said and do not allow yourself to think about something else, however important. Most individuals speak at the rate of 175 to 200 words per minute; however, research suggests that we are very capable of listening and processing words at the rate of 600 to 1000 words per minute. If possible, try to avoid distractions from visitors, phone calls, etc. Be silent, attentive and try hard to appear interested.

Show you are listening

Non-verbal signals show that you are listening, such as maintaining eye contact, nodding, leaning forward. Do not fidget. Communication 'experts' suggest that non-verbal messages can be three times as powerful as verbal messages. Therefore, effective communication becomes difficult if you send non-verbal messages that you're not really listening. Reflect feelings to encourage the speaker to be open.

Don't interrupt

Allow the speaker to finish and don't interrupt.

Don't jump to conclusions

Avoid early judgements about what the speaker is saying or what you anticipate they might say next. As you can listen at a faster rate than most speakers talk, there is a tendency to evaluate too quickly and jump to conclusions. This is perhaps the greatest barrier to effective listening. It is doubly important when listening to a person with whom you disagree. When listeners begin to disagree with a sender's message, they tend to misinterpret the remaining information and distort its intended meaning so that it is consistent with their own beliefs. So maintain an open mind.

Avoid becoming defensive

Don't take what is said personally when what is said is not meant to be personal. Don't become angry; effective listening does not mean that you will have to agree. Too much time spent explaining, elaborating and defending your decision or position is a sure sign that you are not listening because your role has changed from listening to convincing others they are wrong. If you disagree, simply respond with, 'I understand your point. We just disagree on this one.' Effective listeners listen calmly to another person even when that person is offering unjust criticism.

Clarify and summarise

To clarify and summarise by paraphrasing is the art of putting into your own words what you thought you heard and reflecting it back to the sender. For example, a trainee might say: 'You have been unfair to rate me so low on my appraisal.' A paraphrased response might be: 'I can see that you are upset about your appraisal. You think it was unfair.' Paraphrasing is useful because you have to listen very carefully in order to accurately paraphrase and the paraphrasing response will clarify for the sender that their message was correctly received and encourage them to expand on what they are trying to communicate.

Listen to the whole message

Observation is not solely about concentrating on the words being said, but also on the way they are being said. In other words, listen to the whole message. The way a speaker is sitting or standing, the tone of voice and inflection they are using, what the speaker is doing with their hands are all part of the message. A raised voice may be anger or frustration. Looking down while speaking could be embarrassment or shyness. People who make eye contact and lean forward suggest confidence. Arguments may reflect worry. Inappropriate silence may be a sign of aggression.

Check your understanding

Ask questions to make sure you have correctly understood the message being sent, to clarify points or to obtain additional information. Open-ended questions are best, as they require the speaker to convey more information. Frame questions in a way that suggests you have not yet drawn any conclusions. This assures the speaker that not only are you interested but you are looking to obtain more information. The more information that you as listener have, the better you can respond to the sender's communication.

Other

❍ Takes notes where appropriate and with agreement if that seems necessary.
❍ Respect trust and confidences.

Giving feedback

Feedback is part of education and training. Improving you feedback skills will help motivate and develop trainees' knowledge, skills and behaviour. It attempts to identify areas for improvement and actions to be taken to improve them.

It can be informal as in everyday sessions between seniors and trainees, or just between colleagues, or formal as part of written or clinical assessment. However, Ramsden (2003) says 'there is no sharp dividing line between assessment and teaching in the area of giving feedback on learning'. Feedback is part of the overall dialogue between a teacher and learner, not a one-way communication. If there is no feedback the trainee will assume everything is fine and no improvement is required. Many learning opportunities are wasted if they are not accompanied by feedback. Opportunities are also wasted if the learner cannot reflect honestly on their performance. Remember one of the main purposes of feedback is to encourage reflection.

So feedback is essential and the most effective is based on observable behaviours and is practical, timely and concrete. Feedback should be given with sensitivity. Begin by asking the trainee to tell you what they feel confident of doing well and what they would like to improve. Follow up with your observations on what was done well by being specific and then outline one or two points that could help the trainee to improve.

Giving and receiving feedback well requires a high level of skill and confidence that takes time to develop. The Johari window (*see* Chapter 1, section on 'Self-awareness') demonstrates that seeking feedback and disclosing information about ourselves in order to elicit feedback from others has the effect of enlarging the open quadrant. Typically, as I share something about myself (moving information from my hidden quadrant into the open), and if the other party is interested in getting to know me, they will reciprocate, by similarly disclosing information in their hidden quadrant. Thus, an interaction between two parties can be modelled dynamically as two active Johari windows. It helps to choose someone you feel you can trust and whose response will give you some insight into yourself.

As your level of confidence develops, you may actively invite others to comment on your blind spots. You may already seek feedback from students on the quality of a particular lecture, with the desire of improving the presentation. The next stage is to invite comment on your ability to deal with more complex aspects of your role. Self-disclosure – giving the other person something about yourself that helps to build mutual confidence and trust – is an excellent way to start.

Principles of giving effective feedback

Whether you are giving formal or informal feedback, there are a number of basic principles to keep in mind. Personal help can be useful, but sometimes people are hurt by the feedback they receive so be aware of the following.

- Be sensitive to the impact of your message.
- Give feedback only when asked to do so or if your offer to do so is accepted.
- Give feedback as soon after the event as possible.
- Focus on the positive.
- Do it privately wherever possible, especially negative feedback.
- Stay in the 'here and now'; don't bring up previous mistakes, unless this is to highlight a pattern of behaviour.
- Focus on behaviours that can be changed.
- Talk about specifics, giving examples where possible and do not evaluate or assume motives.
- Use 'I' and give your experience of the behaviour ('When you said . . ., I thought that you were . . .').
- When giving negative feedback, suggest alternative behaviours.
- Encourage reflection. This will require open questions such as:
  - What did you learn from this?
  - Did it go as you planned? If not, why not?
  - If you were doing it again, would you do it differently? Why?
  - How did you feel about it? How would you feel about doing it again?
  - How do you think the patient felt? What makes you think that?
- Do not overload; give only two or three key messages.

In Chapter 1 you will find a description of the Kolb learning-style inventory. Giving feedback can be seen as part of this four-stage cycle with feedback supporting the process of reflection.

A number of colleges and deaneries quote Pendleton's Rules, a more structured (and sometimes rigid) approach to providing feedback. After the observed event the following steps are utilised in order.

1 Ask the trainee: 'What do you believe went well?'
2 Offer what you think went well, e.g. 'This is what I think you did well . . .'
3 Ask: 'What would you do differently if you had the opportunity to do it again?"
4 Tell the trainee what you think they might do differently and discuss these points.

Some people point to limitations of these rules by the separation of 'what went well' and the 'what could be done differently', as they can seem artificial. It may appear quite structured and take a long time to identify the learner's needs. One approach is that essentially good feedback should centre on the fundamental principle that it is outcome-based. Therefore the fundamental questions are:

o What were you trying to achieve?
o What were you aiming for?
o What did you try to do to get there?
o What could you have done differently to help you get there?

A number of different models have been developed for giving feedback in a structured and positive way. These include reflecting observations in a chronological fashion; for example, replaying the events that occurred during the session back to the learner. This can be helpful for short feedback sessions, but you can become bogged down in detail during long sessions.

Another model is the 'feedback sandwich', which starts and ends with positive feedback.

When giving feedback to individuals or groups an interactive approach is deemed to be most helpful. This helps to develop a dialogue between the learner and the person giving feedback and builds on the learner's own self-assessment. It is collaborative and helps learners take responsibility for their own learning.

This is not the place to explore the subject fully, but Kurtz and colleagues (2005) devote a chapter in their book to analysing feedback in experiential teaching sessions and for those interested in the subject it is worth a look.

While on the subject of giving feedback, that given to unsuccessful candidates after selection interviews, often regarded as an essential part of the interview process, is discussed more fully later in this chapter in the section on 'Core interviewing skills' (p. 87).

Possible barriers to giving effective feedback

Some are potential barriers and not a great problem if handled with sensitivity and skill, but they may include:

o a trainee who is resistant or defensive when receiving criticism; poor handling of this situation can result in all feedback being disregarded afterwards
o fear of upsetting the trainee
o reluctance to damage the trainee–doctor relationship
o fear of doing more harm than good
o feedback being too generalised and not related to specific facts or observations
o feedback without guidance on how to rectify behaviour
o inconsistent feedback from multiple sources
o a lack of respect for the source of feedback
o lack of sensitivity
o dependent and subordinate position of trainee to trainer (issue of organisational power and authority) and tensions around professional role boundaries and status

o differences in sex, age or educational and cultural background.

Negative feedback

Negative feedback should also be specific and non-judgemental, possibly offering a suggestion: 'Have you thought of . . .?' Focus on some of the positive aspects before considering the areas for improvement.

o 'You maintained eye contact during the consultation. I feel this helped to reassure the patient.'
o 'You picked up most of the key points in the history, including A and B but you did not ask about C.'

Avoid giving negative feedback in front of other people, especially patients. Trainees should be encouraged to seek feedback themselves from others, as feedback actually works best when it is sought.

Giving formal feedback

Perhaps following an appraisal an end of attachment assessment with formal feedback will occur. You may also be required to participate in formal clinical and non-clinical assessments which ideally should incorporate feedback. If feedback has been carried out regularly, the formal feedback sessions should not contain any surprises for the trainee. Feedback can be given on a one-to-one basis or in small groups. The structure for giving feedback needs to be agreed between you and the trainee(s), and may follow one of several models, some of which are described above. It is also important that both you and the subject(s) to whom you are giving feedback are fully prepared for the session.

Prior to a formal feedback session

o Make sure the trainee is aware they are to receive feedback.
o Clearly define the purpose of the feedback session prior to or at the start of the session, collecting any information you need from other people.
o Summarise the feedback.
o Make sure you know the positive aspects and areas for improvement are listed (with supporting evidence).
o Make sure you know how the feedback relates to the learning programme and defined outcomes.

During the formal feedback session

o Agree the purpose and duration of the feedback session.
o Clarify the structure of the session.
o Encourage the learner to self-assess their performance prior to giving feedback.
o Encourage a dialogue and rapport with the trainee.
o Reinforce good practice with specific examples.
o Identify, analyse and explore potential solutions for poor performance or deficits in practice.

After the session
- Complete any outstanding documentation.
- Make sure the learner has copies.
- Carry out any agreed follow-up activities or actions.
- Make sure that opportunities for remedial work or additional learning are arranged.
- Set a date for the next feedback session, if required.

Difficulties with feedback

Sometimes feedback is not received positively by learners and fear of this can inhibit trainers giving regular face-to-face feedback. People's responses to criticism, however constructively it is framed, can vary. Learners often discount their ability to take responsibility for their learning and their responses may present in negative ways, including anger, denial, blaming or rationalisation (King 1999).

When giving feedback, it is helpful to maintain an empathic yet consistent approach with a view to helping the learner take responsibility for development and improvement. It is also helpful to think in a structured way about how feedback might be received. You can help to prepare learners (and yourself) for receiving feedback by providing opportunities for them to practise the guidelines listed below. The aim of developing an open dialogue between the person giving feedback and the recipient is so that both parties are relaxed and able to focus on actively listening, engaging with the learning points and messages and developing these into action points for future development.

Guidelines for receiving constructive feedback

- Listen to the feedback rather than preparing your response/defence.
- Ask for it to be repeated if you did not understand it clearly.
- Assume it is constructive until proven otherwise; then consider and use those parts that are constructive.
- Stop and think before responding.
- Ask for clarification and examples if statements are unclear or unsupported.
- Accept it positively rather than dismissively.
- If not offered, ask for suggestions of ways you might modify or change your behaviour.
- Respect and thank the person giving feedback.

Breaking bad news

As explained above, the development of the skills of communication as a junior doctor is essential but often has to be learnt. Communication is a reciprocal process which enables the exchange of verbal and non-verbal messages between people to convey emotions, information, ideas and knowledge. It also connects the psychological, social and physical domains of patient care. Poor communication is one of the commonest causes of complaint in healthcare; MDU data shows that it is a feature in a large proportion of clinical negligence cases.

The use of such skills is particularly crucial when you have to be the bearer of bad news. It is an unfortunate consequence of working in healthcare that you will be called on from time to time to be the bearer of upsetting information. That news can include any information that changes a patient's, or their loved ones', view of the future in a negative way. In this context bad news can come in many forms for doctors. It may refer to:

○ terminal illness
○ diagnosis of a chronic illness (e.g. diabetes mellitus)
○ disability or loss of function (e.g. impotence)
○ a treatment plan that is burdensome or painful
○ the death of a patient.

Bad news is defined as 'any information that produces a negative alteration to the person's expectations about their present and future' (Fallowfield and Jenkins 2004).

Hippocrates recommended that doctors be wary of breaking bad news because 'the patient may take a turn for the worse'. In *Medical Ethics* for 1803, Thomas Percival gave a similar warning, as did the American Medical Association in its first code of medical ethics in 1847.

In fact, withholding bad news from patients was commonly practised until quite recently. In 1961 a survey of 193 doctors revealed that 169 (88%) routinely withheld cancer diagnoses. Furthermore, they often used euphemisms such as 'growth' to describe cancer. The policy was to tell as little as possible in the most general terms consistent with maintaining co-operation and treatment. The same study revealed that most patients really wanted the truth about their diagnoses. In fact, many recent studies have found that most patients want to know the truth about their illness.

Therefore, a model that emphasizes patient autonomy and full disclosure has replaced a paternalistic model of care. Honest disclosure allows patients to make informed decisions. Withholding bad news diminishes patient autonomy. When a patient eventually realises the nature of their illness he or she may no longer trust the doctor. In fact, good practice now indicates that only under rare circumstances is nondisclosure of bad news ethical.

Breaking bad news can be a difficult task. How it is done may affect patient comprehension of, and acceptance of, the news, to say nothing of their relationship with their doctors. Some of the barriers to effective communication of bad news have been identified as follows:

○ fear of being blamed by the patient
○ not knowing all of the answers sought by the patient or relatives
○ inflicting pain on the patient
○ doctors' personal fears, even their own fear of illness and death
○ little or no formal training in how to break bad news
○ lack of time to give to the task
○ cases with multiple doctors making it unclear who should break the bad news.

Breaking bad news requires expertise, knowledge and skill but also requires compassion.

You should give careful thought to your own perspective on the kinds of issues which will arise for the person receiving the bad news.

The basic principles
Who

The consultant is normally the lead person but does not necessarily need to be the person who does it. Make sure you are clear about what the person is to be told. Remember the recipient may like to have another person with them. This could be a relative or friend, or someone for support, such as a priest or social worker.

Where

Ideally, a specially designated area should be used. In any event, it must be private. An office might suffice but ensure there are no interruptions from people entering, the telephone going or from your pager. Try to arrange for comfortable seating without the barrier of a desk.

How

The use of a breaking bad news model is extremely useful, such as SPIKES, which is a six-step approach.
o **S**etting up the conversation – an appropriate environment, the provision of tissues, allowing the time and avoiding interruptions.
o Assessing the patient's **P**erception of their illness – 'What have you been told already?'
o **I**nviting the patient to disclose information – 'What do you know about your condition?'
o Giving **K**nowledge and information.
o Providing **E**mpathetic support for the emotional response of the patient.
o **S**ummarise and discuss the plans for the future.

Avoid medical jargon. Patients and families will be confused, so don't make it even worse. Be honest; if you do not know something, say so. But let them know if there is someone who does. Check their understanding and when you have finished, make sure there is someone to accompany them after your meeting.

Use appropriate eye contact, voice tone and body language. Remember the old saying: only 7% of the message is in the 'words', there is 55% in the 'dance' and 38% in the 'music'. Ensure that you know what the recipient wants to know and that the time is appropriate for them. All people being told are given the same information, with the same options, including an offer of a second opinion. The information should be factual. Give recipients an opportunity to return for further information or clarification.

Ensure that time is allocated not just to breaking the news but to supporting the recipient. In order to ensure that the patient's GP can deal effectively with them, make sure the GP is informed promptly of what the patient has been told. Your hospital will have a time scale for this, normally within two days. The medical record should be fully updated with notes of your consultation with the patient.

The practicalities

The essentials in preparation are as follows.

o Check the case details thoroughly.
o Make sure you have all information and results to hand.
o Take the notes with you in case you need to refer to them for details.
o Remember that another member of staff present is helpful, not only for you, but to help and support the relative(s).

Your appearance and approach are important. If you wear scrubs, it should go without saying that you should make sure there are no bloodstains, particularly if it is a case of major trauma. Adoption of an appropriate mood can be difficult if one is pressed for time, stressed or unprepared. First check identities and relationships; it is not the time to get names and relationships wrong. Offer your own identity and status and that of anyone with you.

A brief neutral conversation to establish rapport may be beneficial, but do not delay getting on with the purpose of the meeting. You might explain why you have brought someone with you. The reason for meeting should be explained. It is helpful to find out what they already know or have been told; it cannot be assumed that they have previously been prepared for the possibility. Empathise, comfort where necessary, allow time for information to sink in, do not argue and allow relatives their expressions of anger without criticism. Check their understanding, invite questions and try to be practical.

Finally, offer to remain with them for a while in case they wish to ask questions perhaps, although they may wish to be alone. When finished summarise and check what the relatives wish to do immediately. They may wish to see the body. Give them the opportunity to attend to their appearance if they have been crying.

Some further thoughts

There are countless articles and books on this subject and a review of nearly a hundred showed that there are few trials of strategies for breaking bad news. Most writing on the subject is opinion, albeit by experienced practitioners. It is said that the most important factors for individual patients when they receive bad news are the doctor's competence, honesty and attention, the time allowed for questions, a straightforward and understandable diagnosis and the use of clear language. Families rank privacy, the doctor's attitude, competence, clarity and time for questions as important. Knowing the doctor well and the doctor's use of physical contact (for example, by holding the patient's hand) rank lower.

You might sometimes need to get the patient's permission to share bad news, particularly for patients from some non-Western cultures in which autonomy of the individual may not be paramount and healthcare decisions frequently shared with others.

Also, informing patients about possible outcomes before ordering tests or procedures may help prepare patients for potential bad news. You can ask patients if they want only basic information or a detailed disclosure. Remember that although patients need enough information to make informed healthcare decisions, they need to understand. So, for example, the word 'spread' should be used in place of 'metastasised'. Also it is helpful to check frequently that the patient understands, perhaps by asking 'Am I making sense?' or 'Can I clarify anything?' Undue bluntness and misleading optimism should be avoided.

An empathic doctor acknowledges a patient's emotional response to bad news by first identifying the emotion and then responding to it. 'I can see that you are upset by this news' is an empathic statement. Deliberate periods of silence allow patients to process bad news and vent emotions. After receiving bad news, a patient may experience a sense of isolation and uncertainty. Doctors can minimise the patient's anxiety by summarising the areas discussed, checking for comprehension and formulating a strategy and follow-up plan with the patient. Written materials such as hand-written notes, or prepared materials listing the diagnosis and treatment options, may be helpful.

The use of an empathic communication may improve the experience for you and reduce the patient's anxiety. Helpful phrases include:

o 'I wish I had better news' (as opposed to 'I'm sorry, I have bad news.').
o 'I admire your courage.'
o 'I will be here for you.'
o 'What gives you hope and strength?'

Unhelpful statements include:
o 'It could be worse.'
o 'We all die.'
o 'I understand how you feel.'
o 'Nothing more can be done.'

Suggested actions

Ask if you can sit in with someone who is experienced and skilled at breaking bad news.

When you feel confident enough try doing it yourself, maybe with a more experienced person sitting in to help if things get difficult.

Afterwards reflect on what went well and what less well and ask for some feedback from the person who sat in to help.

Only when you feel confident, try doing these interviews on your own.

Complaints and anger

Interpersonal skills are vital in dealing with complaints and these are dealt with in Chapter 6, 'Non-clinical involvement with patients'. Anger management is dealt with in Chapter 4, 'Managing day-to-day issues'.

Core interviewing skills

A great deal of doctors' time is spent in one-to-one meetings, many of which might be described as an interview. They may not always be labelled as such, but each time we need to find out about a patient, the opinions of a colleague, recruit, appraise or discipline a colleague, break bad news or deal with a complaint, we are using inter-viewing skills.

The most important skill related to interviewing is that of questioning. A clear understanding of the use of different types of question is essential. You should remem-ber, however, that getting the words right is only one part of the process. Your manner, tone of voice, facial expression and posture all go together with the words to influence the interviewee's willingness to 'open up'.

Selection interviewing

As with most things in life, interviews are usually much more effective if the panel has put in enough preparation time before the interview starts. Thought should be given to how a panel will work together, what the priorities are for the interviewers, what style of questioning will be used, how the seating should be arranged to put the candidate at ease, and so on. Panel members should have familiarised themselves with the paperwork and have a good idea about what approach they wish to take to questioning the candidates. The role of the chairperson is critical, particularly during the preparation stages that are aimed at getting the panel to work as a team, and then after the interview when the panel is concerned with making the right decision.

Types of questions and their uses

The following approach to using questions to elicit useful information is framed in the context of selection interviewing. The basic approach is transferable to most other interview situations. It helps if you think of interviews as conversations with a purpose. The most effective interviews will generally feel fairly relaxed, if challenging for the interviewee. The aim should be to help them to feel relaxed and prepared to open up about things that perhaps they had not intended.

Behavioural questions

Traditional approaches to medical interviews tended to allow candidates to supply set-piece answers to well-signalled questions, such as 'What do you understand to be the purpose of clinical governance?', or hypothetical questions which only tell the questioner that the interviewee may have a theoretical understanding of the topic, which has probably already been assessed in an examination: 'What would you do if you were faced with . . . ?'

Questions that focus on the interviewee's past experience, their 'real life' events, are generally the most revealing. It is argued that we can understand more about a person's future behaviour by getting to know how they have behaved in the past − 'the best predictor of future behaviour is past behaviour'. This questioning technique requires skill to 'draw out' the interviewee. Questions might start with 'Tell me about your work in . . . ?', or 'Tell us about a situation in which you had to deal with . . . ' The answer is then probed in order to gain insight into the person's past behaviour patterns, motives, values, attitudes and personality. An approach which uses open questions, followed by probing and reflective questions, is most likely to succeed in allowing you to understand the person.

Open questions

Open-ended questions oblige the interviewee to respond with a full answer – they do not permit a 'Yes' or 'No' response. They are likely to start with 'How', 'Why', 'When' or 'Where' or 'Can you tell me about . . . ?' The aim is to get the interviewee to talk to you in their own words so that you can pick up hints that allow you to probe more deeply.

Closed questions

These are useful when checking facts. They are generally phrased to attract a 'Yes' or 'No' response. You may need to be absolutely sure you have the information you need: 'Did you pass the examination?' or 'Was your paper published?' Closed questions can be unhelpful in some cases. In history taking, they may lead patients to give answers that match the doctor's assumptions rather than the patient's real symptoms.

Probing questions

Use probing questions to explore in greater detail actions, experiences and associated opinions and feelings that have been hinted at in the answers to earlier open questions. The candidate will not normally mind gentle interruptions with short questions; for example, 'How did the patient respond to that treatment?', 'How did you feel when they did that?', or 'What did you do then?'

Interruptions are usually acceptable if they are in the form of a probing or deflective question and the interviewer continues to show interest in the interviewee. This approach involves careful listening and some practice if it is to work well.

At the end of a response to an open question it can be effective to pause and allow the interviewee to give more detail or to expand on the last point made. A small gesture may be used, or you may merely add a comment such as: 'And . . . ?' Or 'Go on.'

Silence can also be a very effective way of getting the candidate to open up in areas they had not intended to tell you about. We sometimes feel uncomfortable if a long silence occurs during a conversation. This can lead us to fill it, usually with an ill-thought out and often unhelpful contribution. Silence can have a positive effect in the interview. It can be used to put gentle pressure on the interviewee. This requires a discipline not always found in less experienced interviewers, who must stop themselves from talking while the seconds pass.

Reflective questions

These are for checking understanding, and also serve to elicit further explanation. They involve selecting a word, or a few words, from the interviewee's most recent response and feeding them back as a question: 'You felt unsure?' or: 'You took responsibility for the patient?'

These questions work well in counselling situations, but can also be powerful in getting interviewees in selection or appraisal interviews to go into greater depth regarding their motives and feelings.

Scenario-based questions

This style of questioning is increasingly used in medical interviews, particularly during selection for progression through training. Trainees' responses are graded against predetermined criteria according to how well they answer the question. Examples might include the following.

The surgical trainee candidate might be asked to explain how they would respond if faced with an Anaesthetic Registrar who refuses to anaesthetise a patient for an appendicectomy.

Positive responses might include questioning the Registrar, reflection on the possible reasons for the response such as co-morbidity, the timing during the day, and a review of the decision to operate. More probing questions might be used by the interviewers to elicit an awareness of the patient's need to know what is going on. On the other hand, responses that indicated insistence on proceeding, threatening a critical incident, going over the head of the Registrar and discussing the matter with a senior consultant, or accepting the Registrar's response without questioning it, would be likely to lead to a negative assessment of the candidate.

A clinical example of scenario-based questioning could be based in the A&E department – a 12-year-old boy has fallen off his bicycle. He has a broken arm (supracondylar fracture) and is complaining of breathlessness. The candidate is first asked an open question, such as 'How would you respond to this situation?'

Successful responses would show an awareness of possible vascular injury to the arm; possible pneumothorax and the risk of associated intra-abdominal injury such as a ruptured spleen. The possibility of head injury might also be considered.

Negative assessment would result from responses which failed to take a history of the nature of the accident or the patient's history including possibility of asthma, failure to perform an examination including the trachea, sending patient for CXR without excluding tension pneumothorax, and failing to assess circulation in arm.

Leading questions

Interviewers sometimes try to help the candidate to understand the question by first setting the context for it. The effect is to give the interviewee the answer in the question. These are seldom, if ever, helpful to the interviewer. For example, the interviewer might say: 'We attach a great deal of importance to good teamwork. How do you find you get on in teams?'

It is far better to use the situational approach described above. Ask for the candidate's experience of particular types of work events (e.g. situations they have found stressful), and then try to probe to uncover any successes or problems that have arisen, in particular those that relate to working closely with colleagues.

Feedback to unsuccessful candidates

Giving feedback to unsuccessful candidates who have attended for interview is considered best practice in recruitment and selection. (More detailed discussion on feedback in general is given earlier in this chapter.) An appropriate member of the interview panel should be sought and agree to be responsible for providing feedback that can be an uncomfortable process for the person giving the feedback. Alternatively, each candidate may be allocated a panel member who will if required to give feedback. It is helpful if this person is decided in advance as they can then make notes of helpful feedback points about the candidates during the interview.

Those giving feedback should bear in mind the psychological state of the failed candidates. Most will be upset at having failed to obtain the post so information for feedback should be based on this knowledge. They are likely to be sensitive to strongly adverse criticism. So feedback should be given based on the basis that the person:

- wants feedback
- understands it
- accepts it
- can do something about it.

This can be achieved in the following way.

- Check whether the candidate wants feedback; not everyone does!
- Focus on being constructive by starting with something positive, suggesting ways in which the candidate may improve skills and experience.
- Ensure that the feedback is based on an objective judgement relevant to the person specification.
- Ensure feedback is based on the notes taken during the interview.
- Deal only with a few (one or two) areas for action.
- Concentrate on the highs and lows during the interview by referring to specific behaviour.
- Concentrate on things within the individual's control.
- Do not overload the individual.
- Reference to any knowledge of the candidate that did not form part of the application or selection process must not be made.
- Feedback must be consistent with the decision of the selection panel, even if as provider of feedback you do not agree with the decision.
- Feedback must not be given to anyone except the candidate.
- Feedback must not involve discussion about other candidates.
- A record should be kept of any feedback given to candidates.

If a trainee's serious shortcomings come to light during a selection process, they need to be dealt with through the postgraduate dean or clinical tutor. It is probably not appropriate to bring up such issues at the end of the interview.

Presentation skills

Effective communication of ideas is fundamental to the development of professional knowledge. Postgraduate professional development is partly dependent on doctors sharing research and knowledge with colleagues in regular meetings. Your ability to make effective presentations can also have a significant effect on your career opportunities, since self-presentation is a key factor in attracting attention to your potential.

For the purpose of this section, presentations are taken to mean any situation in which you are required to communicate information, ideas, propositions or a report to an audience of any size. These might include presenting an audit report to a department, reviewing a paper, or contributing to a presentation with others. Making an effective presentation means knowing how to present your ideas, your research and yourself confidently and to the best advantage.

Of course, you want to be able to do this without spending too long agonising over it. This section will help you make the most of your opportunities in making a good impression as a presenter in both formal and informal situations. It will do this by taking you through the processes involved in preparing a good presentation. That is, by:

o selecting relevant material
o organising that material
o delivering it to the best effect.

The first important thing to realise about presentation situations is that, although our basic medium of communication is words, they account for only a small part of the total message. It is generally accepted that less than 25% of what you communicate will be concerned with your words, and some 75% will be concerned with the way you use your voice and with body language, such as facial expression, posture and gestures. You cannot give a good presentation unless you have done the right kind of careful preparation. As part of your preparation you must have the answers to six fundamental questions.

o **Why** am I speaking? What is the purpose of the talk? Is it to inform, to teach, to make a proposition or to inspire and motivate? Defining your objective, preferably in a single sentence, will make preparation simpler and focus the talk.
o **Who** am I speaking to? The size, mix, level of understanding and attitudes of the audience must be taken into account during preparation. Levels of complexity and volume of information and ideas will depend on the likelihood that members of the audience can absorb them in the time available.
o **Where** am I speaking? Always try visiting the venue before your presentation. Check the equipment is working, decide where you will stand and whether your voice will carry without a microphone. Remember that the presence of an audience will deaden the impact and volume of your voice. Make sure the seating layout suits the kind of presentation you have in mind.
o **When** am I speaking? If your presentation is to be made at the end of the working day, you will need to take into account the energy level of members of the audience. The duration of the talk should affect its structure and level of detail. Avoid trying to pack in too much for the audience to absorb in the time available. Audiences will get restless if you run over your allotted time, so keep to your plan. It helps to note the time by which you must finish and to place a watch in front of you at the beginning of your presentation.
o **What** am I going to say? The content will be determined by the objective. Keep returning to your objective statement in order to avoid losing direction. The material is normally organised in one of the following ways:

- a generalisation followed by detailed explanation or illustration
- using a time, spatial or geographical sequence, or a sequence based on ascending or descending order of importance of each element
- contrasting one set of facts/ideas with another
- dividing a unit up into its component parts and saying a little about each.

Ask yourself which method will help you to present your material most effectively, then you are ready to write the first draft. Most good presentations are divided into an introduction, which sets the scene and prepares the audience for what is to come; a main body comprised of three or four main points; and a conclusion, which summarises and emphasises the theme.

- Write your opening and closing sentences in full and learn them 'off by heart'.
- Capture the audience and tell them everything they need to know about the presentation in the opening.
- Make the conclusion really conclusive.

Remember that your presentation will be spoken. When you write your draft, write it in spoken English, not written English. This will help you to sound more natural, even when you are actually reading whole phrases or sentences from your cue cards (as most speakers do from time to time).

To help you achieve a clear, natural style, remember these tips.

- Use simple, familiar words that come to you naturally.
- Only use technical jargon that your audience will understand.
- Use short sentences.

○ **How** am I going to say it? Most speakers use notes or prompt cards, but speak from brief notes to avoid reading word for word. The use of voice and gesture as well as audiovisual aids requires careful thought, practice and self-awareness. For speaking notes:
   - use small cards rather than sheets of paper as they're easier to hold and look more professional
   - write key sentences and key words on the cards
   - fasten the cards together, or at least number them in sequence in case you drop them.

Effective delivery

Paying attention to articulation, pace, intonation and emphasis achieve effective delivery.

○ Good articulation can be achieved by practising enunciation in front of a mirror. Many speakers are 'lazy' in the way they form their sounds, not moving their lips and tongue enough. Keep your head up. Don't speak with your chin down in your collar.

○ Pace should be varied to maintain interest. Nervous speakers always speak too quickly. Avoid racing! Pauses can be used for effect, but they also allow the listeners to absorb the points you are making and react to them.

○ Intonation is the rhythm and inflection in the voice. Most people use only two or three tones of the musical scale when they speak. The Welsh and the Western Highlanders, on the other hand, use about an octave and a half. Get colour into your voice.

○ Emphasis, often coupled with repetition, is a most useful speaking device. If your voice lacks colour, practise emphasising key words and phrases from your cue cards. Remember that you can also emphasise points by using appropriate (but not distracting) gestures.

In general, try to achieve the following.

○ Speak as naturally and conversationally as possible.

○ Stand in a comfortable position with your feet slightly apart.

○ Smile and be friendly.

○ Maintain good eye contact with the whole audience.

○ Check whether you have any distracting mannerisms and work to get rid of them. These may include excessive use of certain phrases or sounds ('space fillers') such as 'you know', 'um', 'er' or 'You see'. Habits such as jingling keys or coins in a pocket, or pacing up and down like a caged tiger, can also be a barrier to effective communication with the audience.

Visual aids

Good use of visual aids will improve your presentation by helping your audience to remember what you have said more easily than if you use words alone. Visual aids used badly or carelessly can be very distracting and even irritating, and are often worse than none at all. PowerPoint is normally regarded as the most professional way to present, but avoid overdoing it. Too many slides and too much use of special effects can be distracting and even irritating for an audience.

○ Check that equipment is in the right place and working properly before you begin.

○ Be sure that everything is large enough to be seen by everyone in the room.

○ Don't read from visuals – you insult the audience's intelligence.

○ Face the audience, not the screen. If you have one, place your laptop so that you can glance at it from time to time.

○ Each picture should have only one main message. Complex slides confuse and bore.

○ Minimise the words on each visual. A maximum of 20 is a good rule of thumb.

○ Words should be in a clear, readable font (in roman not italic), and at least 20-point font size should be used.

○ Always be prepared with back-up material, to cope if the machinery breaks down.

Handouts are sometimes used to support a presentation. It can sometimes be unhelpful to circulate them at the start of your presentation, as they may become a distraction. On the other hand, many people like to have a copy of the presentation so that they can add notes to it as you speak. You should adapt your approach to suit the audience.

Taking questions

o Decide whether you will take questions during or after your presentation and tell your audience your decision clearly in the introduction to your presentation.
o Listen carefully to the question and check that you've understood it.
o Repetition of the question also helps everyone in the room to know exactly what is being answered.
o Do not expect questions to come as soon as you stop talking. You are expecting the audience to go into a different mode, so be prepared to wait or 'plant' a question in the audience to get things going.
o Keep your answers short as you may bore the rest of the audience.

Action

Bearing in mind the above notes, describe in the space below what you see as your strengths and weaknesses as a presenter. If possible seek pointers from a colleague or friend who has seen you make presentations.

Strengths:

Weaknesses:

Now reflect on these, considering which of your weaknesses could be due to lack of experience or learning, and which are unchangeable. Seek to describe them in ways that help you to decide what improvements you need to make in your approach.

Now identify the types of situation in which you expect to make presentations over the next year or so.

At your next presentation, ask a couple of members of the audience (preferably friends who you can rely on to give you helpful feedback) to make notes about the way you make your presentation and tell you what they thought of it afterwards. You and they may find the checklist in Box 3.1 useful as a guide. Do not mention your perceived weaknesses to them beforehand, but quiz them about these aspects of your presentation when you get your feedback.

Good luck!

BOX 3.1 Presentation feedback sheet

Content

Introduction
- Was the purpose clear?
- Was a link made with the audience?
- Did the speaker make an impact within the first two minutes?

Main body
- Was the talk pitched at a level to suit the audience?
- Were there clear stages?
- Did it follow a logical sequence?

Conclusions
- Was there a summary of key points?
- (If relevant) was there an indication of action to be taken, and by whom?

Voice
- Volume too loud/soft?
- Tone varied to maintain interest?
- Pace too fast/slow?

Timing
- Started and finished on time?

Stance
- Relaxed posture, facing audience?

Mannerisms
- Free from distraction, such as pacing, verbal habits?

Visual aids
- Relevant/simple and clear/technically proficient?

Contributing to meetings

There are many different kinds of meeting, including small group, support, events, clinical, staff, departmental, open or public, committees, workshops, learning sessions, conferences and so on. Meetings are a feature of professional life. They are a common event for clinicians representing colleagues, nurse managers and business managers.

They are also expensive and can waste time; for example, when there is no clear objective to the meeting, or a lack of effective leadership and control, or there are too many or the wrong participants. Time is often wasted on debate about 'Why?' rather than 'How?' In addition, a lack of clarity on outcomes produces unclear final decisions or even no decisions. Meetings that do not achieve results not only waste time but also often lead to more meetings.

Aims, planning, teamwork

Every well-run meeting, whether formal or informal, should be based on three prerequisites:

○ clear aims
○ careful planning
○ effective teamwork.

Clear aims should be related to the purpose of the meeting. A departmental meeting may be for talking, listening and sharing problems. A committee normally aims to make and agree decisions, whereas a learning session is about sharing ideas through teaching and learning.

Always go to meetings knowing what you want to achieve.

Advance preparation is vital, and that applies to all participants. How often have you been at a presentation of a new idea and when participants have been asked to comment, nearly everyone has suggestions for improvements? Yet no one was given the opportunity to study the proposal in advance, everyone was seeing it for the first time. Discussions are lengthy and suggestions numerous.

Other time-wasters include fighting losing or lost battles by discussing items decided elsewhere or that are not within the group's power to decide.

Some reasons for meetings

Meetings can be called for all sorts of reasons other than reaching a decision, and these can be classified as follows:

○ creating and developing ideas (e.g. brainstorming sessions)
○ sharing out work and responsibility – usually valuable for small groups only
○ delegation of work or authority within a group
○ sharing responsibility for a difficult problem
○ providing or receiving information – there may be better ways
○ persuasion – best done before the meeting
○ networking, which become 'talking shops'
○ an alternative to preparing a short written report

o committees in the habit of meeting without a real purpose, even with lengthy agendas

o socialising – acceptable at the beginning of a meeting, but do keep it short

o perhaps as a substitute for work.

Decision making at meetings

Decision making on tasks or issues may be a valid reason for calling a meeting, but you need to ask yourself if it is:

o consulting before a decision is made

o gathering information for a decision to be made elsewhere

o gaining agreement on a decision

o seeking a decision that requires the agreement of more than one group

o enhancing commitment to a decision

o making a decision.

Why go to a meeting?

Any meeting you attend is your meeting too. Do you know why you're going? At every meeting you should have a personal objective(s).

Planning for a meeting

Make sure you are fully prepared; otherwise you are failing to be an effective member. It may be the opportunity to put across a message. A seed sown today might be important for later. You can often turn someone else's question into a bridge for your own message. A question directed at you, in any situation, will always give you an opportunity to say what you want. Always answer the question and then make your point. If you are asked a question and you don't know the answer it is perfectly acceptable to say 'I don't know but I'll find out and let you know' and then go on to your statement, via a suitable link. You can also use the same technique in response to a statement, by agreeing with that statement, before linking to your own statement. Here the speaker becomes the leader and controls the meeting while speaking. This is observable at medical committees.

Seating arrangements

Semicircles are good for problem-solving meetings and provide a good balance of control and sensitivity for the leader. Long tables are control mechanisms and inhibit brainstorming sessions. It is impossible to see others down the same side of the table, and discussions between participants are limited. The more eye contact and the more people it is made with, the more control you have.

To some extent where you sit will depend on your purpose. If you want to be uninvolved pick a position that permits that. If you are seeking to win a point or plan seizing control, pick a controlling position. At a long table this will be at either end. At a three-sided arrangement this will be either side of the chair or at either end. At a long table, an ally at the other end of the table will give you maximum support in handling a difficult meeting.

Next time you are at a meeting observe where people sit and see how it influences their roles. If you are going to be a competitor to the chair, sit as far away as possible. The ideal position is opposite, so that you can talk directly to the chair and include others as well.

General meeting techniques

Interruptions

Knowing when to interrupt to gain control is a useful tool. Asking a question is a useful way of interrupting and changing the direction of the meeting. Always maintain a moderate tone and remember that the greatest impact you have will be through your non-verbal communication.

- 'Have you considered . . . ?'
- 'Could I add . . . ?' and continue speaking.
- Call the person by name, 'John, don't forget . . . ', and continue speaking.
- Just start speaking and raise your voice above the level of the other person.

Do not wait for permission to be granted before you interrupt, but continue talking. It is often difficult to hang back while someone presents something that you consider inappropriate. But do think twice before making yourself vulnerable by interrupting the speaker, as your own point may not be quite as perfect as you thought.

If you want to prevent yourself being interrupted:

- insist on finishing by saying: 'Please, just let me finish . . . ' and continue
- hold your hand up, palm outwards, and continue.

Criticism

If your suggestion should be the subject of criticism, ask the critic to present an analysis of your proposal with workable alternatives for the next meeting. Emotion can resist logic. When someone is emotionally aroused, your best ploy is to remain silent until their emotion peters out.

Opposition

When you are up against opposition your objective should always be to determine your opponent's objectives. There is nothing wrong with having a different objective. Ask yourself what your opponent wants and why they want it. Better still, ask them. Only when you know your opponent's priorities can you plan your own strategy.

Confrontation

If you are disagreeing with someone, try to provide your opponent with a way out, a way to save face. If you disagree, first state what you agree with, thus supporting their position as modified by your own. Make criticism less personal by claiming you are acting as the 'devil's advocate'.

Contribute early

Research indicates that when a person contributes early in a discussion, they are likely to exert a greater influence throughout the discussion. Asking questions for clarification or to challenge assumptions is a positive way to contribute at an early stage. This will help you to establish where others stand before committing yourself. This also obliges others to respond to you, but be prepared to come back into the discussion to combat opposing arguments.

Conducting meetings

If you hold the role of chairman or secretary to a regular meeting, you should ask yourself whether the meeting is necessary, and always question the value of minutes as compared with action points. The latter tend to be much easier and quicker to produce, are specific about who is responsible for actions and by which date they should be completed. They can normally be agreed at the end of the meeting. Keeping detailed minutes of meetings means that much time at the beginning of the following meeting is taken up in checking them for accuracy and discussing matters arising. This ritual often wastes time, as matters of real importance are normally dealt with in the meeting agenda. Of course, there are sometimes statutory reasons for maintaining detailed meetings. Occasionally, it is deemed necessary for clinical governance purposes. You should always be prepared to challenge the need for them, however.

A further point to consider is whether the discussion of 'any other business' serves a useful purpose. This item frequently allows those who are too lazy or disorganised to prepare properly for the meeting by submitting agenda items in advance to address their issues when everyone is anxious to leave. This can allow important matters to be inadequately addressed by the meeting. 'Any other business' can also be a golden opportunity for time-wasters to hold up progress on more important matters. Many meetings are conducted without redress to 'AOB' and are considered to be the better for it.

Action

There is an important difference between a stimulating discussion and a productive meeting. For the next meeting you attend, ask yourself the following questions.
- What is the purpose of this meeting?
- What should I achieve by the end?
- How will I distinguish my success from failure?

After the meeting ask the following.
- Was I correct about the task?
- Were the other participants clear about the task and objectives?
- Did I achieve the meeting's objective as stated in the agenda?
- Was the meeting a success or failure?
- If it was a failure, why?

- What could be done to improve the next meeting?
- What was done that should be discontinued?
- What could the chairperson do to improve the meeting?
- Could you have done without the meeting?
- If so, how?

Being interviewed

Before considering interviews, it might be worth reflecting on the importance of your CV or application as a basis for, firstly, being short-listed and, secondly, for the panel to prepare questions. You should remember that at least some of the panel will never have met you, so their first impressions will be coloured by the quality of your application.

Modernising Medical Careers has introduced a more structured, centralised process of recruitment to the appointment of trainees. Deanery-based selection panels deal mostly with applications forms for specialist training posts, but many candidates for interview are still asked to bring copies of their CV to the interview. In some cases, though, application forms are the only source of information for the short-listing panels. CVs may still be required for trust posts or senior medical appointments. The MMC website carries updated information related to the selection process for the different training specialties. The selection process is structured around the person specification, with which you should be wholly familiar before the interview.

Selection interviews for specialist training posts are normally comprised of a number of interviews and assessments. These may involve attendance for at least half a day and may include a traditional interview, a scenario-based interview (*see* above, p. 90), an interview based on the trainee's portfolio and possibly competence tests such as patient simulation exercises.

Prepare everything the day before and allow plenty of time by arriving early and having all possible questions and your answers totally revised and memorised. You need to convince the panel that you will achieve your goals or, in the case of a consultant appointment, make a delightful colleague.

Apart from specialist training appointments, the size of appointment committees tends to grow in relation to the seniority of appointment, although there are guidelines and statutory regulations for the composition of selection committees. In the case of consultant interviews, it is not uncommon for the main interview process to be enhanced by a series of smaller interviews with small groups (say three or four persons) from the multidisciplinary team. These are used to help other future colleagues to have a say in who they will be working with, as well as giving you greater insight into the culture of the organisation. Apart from consultants within a specialty, members of the main selection committee will not all know one another. You can be reassured that even some of the panel members may feel in strange surroundings, and many panel members also confess privately to some nervousness.

As a general rule you should dress to reassure and fit the stereotype of the post for which you have applied. Go into the room positively, smiling and determined to enjoy it. It will not be as bad as a viva examination. Try to:

○ be relaxed but business-like
○ sit upright
○ be friendly, smile with perhaps a degree of authority
○ look initially at the chairperson, who should put you at your ease
○ show enthusiasm for the job.

Interview questions

Routine questions (usually from the chair) about your journey or finding the place help to 'break the ice' and are usually followed by some more routine questions to clarify any queries with your CV, such as unusual features or gaps. The questions then tend to move on to asking you your reasons for wanting the job or what attracted you to it. This is an opportunity to show that you have researched the hospital. Perhaps you have identified a significant challenge that the institution faces. Take care to avoid appearing critical of the trust or its management; they are unlikely to warm to someone who hardly knows them and who finds fault.

The next questions are likely to explore your future career direction. Be enthusiastic and do not give evasive answers. The questions are usually fairly straightforward, and simply aimed at getting you to talk about yourself. Do so with a mixture of confidence, enthusiasm, honesty and maturity as appropriate to the question (it is as easy as that!).

Always address your answer initially to the questioner but look around and try to engage all the panel members with your answer. Be neither monosyllabic nor loquacious; balance is important. Even if asked closed questions, avoid the temptation to give simple 'Yes' or 'No' answers. Try to expand the answer to allow the interviewer time to recover. You will gain no friends by making him or her feel uncomfortable.

The panel will normally have agreed in advance to split up questions into a number of areas, each covered by one panel member. You might be asked about your vision for the hospital and department, what you think of the hospital, or what you have to offer. Typical questions ask about research you have done or intend to do, your experience of clinical audit, government reports that affect you, and the NHS generally, as well as possible future plans and changes in the NHS.

There may be questions that seek to reveal 'what makes you tick'. These are usually about hobbies and outside interests. Avoid suggesting these might interfere with your work! Aptitudes and outside interests are a measure of whether you are a well-rounded personality.

Talking about strengths and weaknesses

The interviewers may try to reveal your virtues and weaknesses, perhaps by asking about your mistakes or weakness directly, or your aptitudes and ambitions. Answers tend to reveal your personal values. Questions about weaknesses, mistakes, tasks that you could have done better, or opportunities missed gauge your self-awareness, intellectual honesty, maturity and dependability, and may relate indirectly to your team-membership characteristics.

There are no right answers to these questions, but it is worth thinking in advance about mistakes you have made, difficult situations you have been in, and times when you have felt out of your depth and how you coped, and what you learned from these experiences.

Pressure questions about previous failed interviews may also give clues about your ability to cope with stress, your maturity and your emotional stability.

Questions about your greatest achievements, challenges or responsibilities are an attempt to obtain a record of your standards, your qualities of management and relationships, as well as your leadership style and ability, and whether you are a process- or people-oriented person. Questions about relationships are trying to assess relationships with colleagues by view of personality: social or self-contained; conforming or independent; extrovert or sensitive; phlegmatic or excitable.

Handling difficult panel members

These are the ones who ask tricky questions that are intended to impress the committee with the questioner's skill. If you are asked that sort of question, stay calm, and if you find you are struggling remember that only better candidates get asked difficult questions to separate them, and that committee members usually have sympathy for candidates being given a difficult time by colleagues.

Handling silence

If there is silence after your answer, you are being invited to continue. Do not be embarrassed by silence, even if you need time to think about your answer. Allow yourself time to think before answering, so that your replies are considered and logical. Do not be tempted to leap in and say something ill-considered.

You need not be embarrassed to have a question clarified if you are not clear what you are being asked, but do not waste time looking for hidden catches. Remember the interviewers are usually seeking reassurance. Do make sure you are answering the question asked. With multiple questions try to remember the individual questions or clarify before answering.

Conclusion

Try to appear friendly, cheerful and smiling. Body language helps with a businesslike authoritative attitude, professional appearance and energetic approach. At the end of the interview you are generally invited by the chair to ask the panel any questions you might have. While it will not count against you to ask a question, it is acceptable and possibly desirable not to do so.

Panel presentations

This is a developing method of helping to assess candidates for consultant appointments, and is thought to be a reasonable way of assessing the vision of candidates in relation to the future of a unit. Whether the candidate has grasped the problems of the unit in pre-interview visits and has a realistic expectation of what they are coming to will also be apparent. Some candidates like it as a way of being in control of the first part of the interview, whereas others feel uncomfortable making presentations, particularly as it will not usually be a part of their everyday work. It does illustrate the importance of making sure you collect useful information from the clinical director, medical director, chief executive and chairperson when paying your pre-application visit.

Related reading

Ariyasena H, Tewari N, Livesley PJ. The search for the perfect curriculum vitae. *BMJ Careers.* 2005; **331**: 167–9.

Barker A. *How to Manage Meetings.* London: Kogan Page; 2007.

BMA. *Communication Skills Education for Doctors: an update, November 2004.* London: British Medical Association; 2004. Available online at: www.bma.org.uk/images/communication _tcm41–20207.pdf

Bradbury A. *Successful Presentation Skills.* London: Kogan Page; 2000.

Fallowfield L, Jenkins V. Communicating sad, bad, and difficult news in medicine. *Lancet.* 2004; **363**: 312–19.

Ghosh R. The consultant interview: secrets to success. *BMJ Careers.* 18 March 2008.

GMC. *Good Medical Practice.* London: General Medical Council; 2006. Available online at: www.gmc-uk.org/static/documents/content/GMC_GMP.pdf

Gray C. Fair interviewing is harder than it looks. *BMJ Career Focus.* 2005; **331**: 68–9.

ICM. *Patients Redress Survey.* ICM; 2002. Available online at: www.icmresearch.co.uk/ reviews/2002/patients-redress-survey.htm

King J. Giving feedback. *BMJ.* 1999; **318**: 2. Available online at: www.bmj.com/cgi/content/ full/318/7200/S2-7200

Kurtz SM, Silverman J, Draper J. *Teaching and Learning Communication Skills in Medicine.* 2nd ed. Oxford: Radcliffe Publishing; 2005.

Maguire P, Pitceathly C. Key communication skills and how to acquire them. *BMJ.* 2002; **325**: 697–700.

MDU Data and Communication Skills. *The MDU 2010 Communication Skills for Doctors Workshops.* Available online at: www.the-mdu.com/section_Hospital_doctors_and_specialists/ topnav_Our_services_5/nav_Education_and_Training_4/subnav_Communication_Skills_ Workshop_2.asp

MMC. *A Reference Guide for Postgraduate Specialty Training in the UK (the Gold Guide).* 3rd ed. London: Modernising Medical Careers; 2009.

Picard O, Wood D, Yuen S. *Medical Interviews: a comprehensive guide to CT, ST and Registrar interview skills.* London: ISC Medical; 2008.

Ramirez AJ *et al.* Mental health of hospital consultants: the effects of stress and satisfaction at work. *The Lancet.* 1996; **347**: 724–8.

Ramsden P. *Learning to Teach in Higher Education.* 2nd ed. Abingdon: Routledge; 2003.

Reynolds P, Harrison M. Consultant interviews are different. *BMJ Career Focus.* 2005; **331**: 73.

Scottish Executive. *Our National Health: a plan for action, a plan for change.* 2000. Available online at: www.scotland.gov.uk/Publications/2000/12/7770/File-1

Scottish Executive. *Talking Matters: developing the communication skills of doctors.* 2003. Available online at: www.scotland.gov.uk/Publications/2003/11/18452/28575#6

Smith C, Meeking D. *How to Succeed at the Medical Interview.* Oxford: Blackwell; 2008.

Managing day-to-day issues

The aim of this chapter is to develop your awareness of a range of aspects for dealing with people at work, resolving conflict, dealing with opposition, acting assertively, dealing with anger, delegation and influencing others, as well as handling stress and helping you to manage your time effectively. It provides some information for developing your skills in leadership and team working, although you cannot learn to lead and influence others just by reading a book – but it can help if you have some background knowledge. Much of this chapter is useful reading for related training workshops.

Leadership

A Medical Leadership Competency Framework (MLCF)

Jointly developed by The AMRC and NHS III, this framework describes the leadership competencies doctors need in order to become more actively involved in the planning, delivery and transformation of health services. It can be used to:

- help design training curricula and development programmes
- highlight individual strengths and development areas through self-assessment and structured feedback from colleagues
- help with personal development planning and career progression.

It is built on the concept of shared leadership where leadership is not restricted to those who hold designated leadership roles and where there is a shared sense of responsibility for the success of the organisation and its services. Acts of leadership can come from anyone in the organisation as appropriate and at different times. They can be focused on the achievement of the group rather than the individual. Therefore shared leadership actively supports effective teamwork.

According to Tooke (2008):

> The doctor's frequent role as head of the healthcare team and commander of con-siderable clinical resource requires that greater attention is paid to management and leadership skills regardless of specialism. An acknowledgement of the leadership role of medicine is increasingly evident. Role acknowledgement and aspiration to enhanced roles be they in sub-specialty practice, management and leadership, educa-tion or research are likely to facilitate greater clinical engagement.

Darzi (2008) added: 'Greater freedom, enhanced accountability and empowering staff are necessary but not sufficient in the pursuit of high-quality care. Making change actually happen takes leadership. It is central to our expectations of the healthcare professionals of tomorrow.' You can download the MLCF document at www.institute. nhs.uk/images/documents/BuildingCapability/Medical_Leadership/Medical%20 Leadership%20Competency%20Framework%202nd%20ed.pdf.

GMC and leading teams

Healthcare is increasingly provided by multidisciplinary teams. This can bring benefits to patient care but problems may arise when communication is poor or responsibilities are unclear. If you manage a team, you will need to recognise when it is not functioning well and know where to go for help.

When leading a team the GMC state you should pay attention to the following.

- Respect the skills and contributions of your colleagues.
- Don't make unfounded criticisms of colleagues which can undermine patients' trust in the care provided.
- Ensure that colleagues understand the professional status and specialty of all team members, their roles and responsibilities in the team and who is responsible for each aspect of patient care.
- Ensure that staff are clear about their individual and team objectives, their personal and collective responsibilities for patient and public safety and for openly and hon-estly recording and discussing problems.
- Communicate effectively with colleagues within and outside the team.
- Make sure that arrangements are in place for relevant information to be passed on to the team promptly.
- Make sure that all team members have an opportunity to contribute to discussions and that they understand and accept the decisions taken.
- Encourage team members to co-operate and communicate effectively with each other.
- Make sure that each patient's care is properly co-ordinated and managed and that patients are given information about whom to contact if they have questions or concerns; this is particularly important when patient care is shared between teams.
- Set up and maintain systems to identify and manage risks in the team's area of responsibility.

○ Monitor and regularly review the team's performance and take steps to correct deficiencies and improve quality.

○ Deal openly and supportively with problems in the conduct, performance or health of team members through effective and well-publicised procedures.

○ Make sure that your team and the organisation have the opportunity to learn from mistakes.

Leading teams

Doctors usually work as part of a team and as your professional status and clinical responsibility grows so does your need to lead and direct others. Leadership is about building relationships, setting goals and achieving results through others. Theories and models of leadership are many and varied. There is no simple or correct approach but many variables that might influence the approach a leader should take to a particular situation. It helps, however, to have insight into some of the established thinking regarding leadership.

Broadly, the development of leadership thinking over the past two centuries has moved through the following stages (Crainer 1996).

○ **Great man theories** are based on the belief that leaders are exceptional people who are born with a propensity and capability to lead in any circumstances. This belief has been pretty well demolished by experience and research, although there are still some who may believe in the idea.

○ **Trait theories** are associated with the assumption that successful leaders exhibit a range of qualities or traits that enable them to do the right thing at the right time. It has proven virtually impossible to isolate a consistent set of traits despite extensive research into the characteristics of well-known successful leaders such as Gandhi and Churchill. One or two do seem to be evident – they are all good communicators, have a vision that followers find attractive and are generally of above-average intelligence (although not super-intelligent). Beyond this there are many inconsistencies that are difficult to resolve.

○ **Power and influence approaches** assume the centralisation of decision making, the exercise of power resulting from this centralisation and passivity in subordinates.

○ **Behaviourist theories** focus on what leaders actually do rather than their innate qualities. Sets of behaviours are categorised and described as different styles.

○ **Situational leadership** sees the leadership process as being determined by the context in which it is carried out. For example, leadership in the field of battle or operating theatre may be different from that in a general practice or high street shop. **Contingency theory** also assumes that the situational variables are the basis for determining best leadership practice.

○ **Transactional theory** emphasises the importance of the relationship between the leader and followers. It is based on a concept of mutual benefit deriving from a form of contract through which the leader delivers rewards and recognition and the followers provide effort, commitment and loyalty.

○ **Attribution theory** emphasises the power of the followers, who assume their role as followers and thus attribute the leadership role to a particular person.
○ **Transformational theory** is grounded in the concept that leadership is all about change and the leader achieves change through creating a vision and sharing this with the followers – this requires a complex set of qualities, skills and capabilities that enable the leader to achieve alignment between team members and the goals of the organisation.

Many of these approaches are merged into contemporary models. Some of the more relevant examples are explored in greater detail below.

Do you (have to) possess the right personality traits?

A traditional view of leadership held that a few people were born with special powers and aptitudes that made them natural leaders. These included enthusiasm, self-assurance, initiative, intelligence and so on. Studies of effective leaders have raised doubts about this view, research having failed to identify a consensus on such traits, particularly because there are many notably successful leaders who are deficient in a significant proportion of the defined traits. However, a few characteristics do seem to be fairly consistent. These include a clear vision that followers understand and are attracted to; for example, the ability to communicate effectively and being of above-average intelligence. While recognising the importance of personal qualities, more attention is now directed to the behaviour and competence of leaders rather than their inherent personal characteristics. Leadership is a complex process that involves a range of skills and qualities which, given aptitude, may be acquired or developed through learning and practice.

Is leadership a matter of style?

Styles of leadership are usually defined as ranging between 'authoritarian' and 'democratic'. The difference between one style and another can sometimes reflect the power relationship between the leader and the led. Authoritarian leaders have power and hold on to it, using it to direct and control the work behaviour of their subordinates. They retain the right to make decisions, to reward and punish. More democratic styles lead to the delegation of decision making or at least to sharing authority and control.

Some writers argue that people are more productive when working in a democratic environment. They reason that supportive styles of leadership help to create job satisfaction, reduce grievance rates and result in less inter-group conflict. Some doubt, however, that such participative styles of leadership are always effective in enhancing group performance. Sometimes circumstances demand a directive style, such as in life-or-death situations. There may also be circumstances when team members are unfamiliar with the task or with working together in a team. Here it may be necessary for a more directive style until the team has matured sufficiently to be able to manage without needing direction from a team leader. Style alone is generally insufficient as a determining factor in success, although it is important.

The following questionnaire helps you to identify your own style. When completing it try to place yourself in a situation in which you might have to lead even if this is not your normal role.

Task/process leadership questionnaire
Source: Pfeiffer and Jones (1974) – used with permission.

The objective of the questionnaire is to identify your leadership style through your relative concern for tasks or people, and locate it in terms of three types of leadership: individual, group or shared.

Directions
The following items describe some aspects of leadership behaviour. Respond to each item according to the way you would be most likely to act if you were the leader of a team or group. You could think of yourself in a group at work, or in a social, hobby or sports group with a job or task to carry out.
    Circle whether you would most likely behave in the described way:

always **(A)**, frequently **(F)**, occasionally **(O)**, seldom **(S)**, or never **(N)**

1	I would most likely act as the spokesperson for a group.	A	F	O	S	N
2	I would encourage people to stay late to finish a task.	A	F	O	S	N
3	I would allow team members complete freedom in the way they worked.	A	F	O	S	N
4	I would encourage team members to use standard procedures.	A	F	O	S	N
5	I would allow people to use their judgement in solving problems.	A	F	O	S	N
6	I would stress trying to be ahead of competing groups.	A	F	O	S	N
7	I would speak as representative of the group.	A	F	O	S	N
8	I would nag members for greater effort.	A	F	O	S	N
9	I would try out new ideas.	A	F	O	S	N
10	I would let people do their work the way they think best.	A	F	O	S	N
11	I would work hard to get praise.	A	F	O	S	N
12	I would tolerate delay and uncertainty.	A	F	O	S	N
13	I would speak for the group if there were outsiders present.	A	F	O	S	N
14	I would keep the work moving at a rapid pace.	A	F	O	S	N
15	I would let people loose on a job and allow them to get on with it.	A	F	O	S	N
16	I would settle any conflicts if they occurred.	A	F	O	S	N
17	I would get swamped with details.	A	F	O	S	N
18	I would represent the group at outside meetings.	A	F	O	S	N

always **(A)**, frequently **(F)**, occasionally **(O)**, seldom **(S)**, or never **(N)**

19	I would be reluctant to allow the group any freedom of action.	A	F	O	S	N
20	I would decide what should be done and how it should be done.	A	F	O	S	N
21	I would push for maximum effort.	A	F	O	S	N
22	I would let some people have control which I could have kept.	A	F	O	S	N
23	Things usually turn out as I predict.	A	F	O	S	N
24	I would allow people a high degree of initiative.	A	F	O	S	N
25	I would assign people to particular tasks.	A	F	O	S	N
26	I would be happy to make changes.	A	F	O	S	N
27	I would ask people to work harder.	A	F	O	S	N
28	I would trust the group members to exercise their judgement.	A	F	O	S	N
29	I would arrange how the work was to be done.	A	F	O	S	N
30	I would not explain my reasons.	A	F	O	S	N
31	I would persuade team members of the advantages of my ideas.	A	F	O	S	N
32	I would allow the group to set their own pace.	A	F	O	S	N
33	I would urge my group to better their previous efforts.	A	F	O	S	N
34	I would not consult the group.	A	F	O	S	N
35	I would ask that people used only approved methods.	A	F	O	S	N

P = _____   **T** = _____

Scoring the questionnaire is reasonably straightforward as long as you follow the instructions below step by step.

Scoring is as follows:

1 Circle the item number for items 8, 12, 17, 18, 19, 30, 34 and 35.
2 Write the number 1 in front of a *circled item number* if you responded **S** (seldom) or **N** (never) to that item.
3 Also write a number 1 in front of *item numbers not circled* if you responded **A** (always) or **F** (frequently).
4 Circle the number 1s which you have written in front of the following items: 3, 5, 8, 10, 15, 18, 19, 22, 24, 26, 28, 30, 32, 34 and 35.
5 *Count* the *circled number* 1s. This is your score for concern for people. Record the score in the blank following the letter **P** at the end of the questionnaire.
6 *Count the uncircled number* 1s. This is your score for concern for tasks. Record this number in the blank following the letter **T**.

Now follow the instructions below to plot your **T–P** leadership style profile.

To determine your style of leadership, mark your score on the concern for task dimension (**T**) on the left-hand arrow in Figure 4.1.

Next, move to the right-hand arrow and mark your score on the concern for people dimension (**P**).

Draw a straight line that intersects the **P** and **T** scores. The point at which the line crosses the shared leadership arrow indicates your position on that dimension.

A high score on the **T** dimension and a low **P** score indicates a strong tendency to focus on getting the job done, perhaps at the expense of maintaining good working relations with the team. High **P** and low **T** probably means that team members are at ease with your style, although they might prefer to get more direction at times, even at the expense of having an easy time. The higher your score on the middle (shared) dimension, the more you are likely to be able to adjust your style to suit situations where either a 'telling' style is more appropriate, or to one in which you involve the team in the decision making.

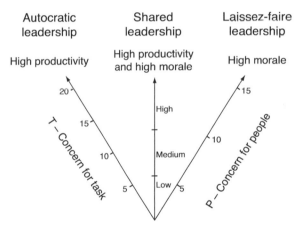

FIGURE 4.1 Shared leadership results from balancing concern for task and concern for people

Leadership style is partly about taking into account the situation!

By taking into account the situation, 'effective' leaders get the task done while maintaining good working relationships with their colleagues and within the team. Appropriate leadership style is about finding a balance between task-oriented and relationship-oriented leadership behaviour.

o **Task-oriented behaviour** focuses on directing the actions of others, defining roles, setting goals and giving clear direction.
o **Relationship-oriented behaviour** concerns the extent to which the leader engages in listening, encouraging and supporting group members both as individuals and as members of a team.

It is these two dimensions that produce the five leadership styles set out in Figure 4.2.

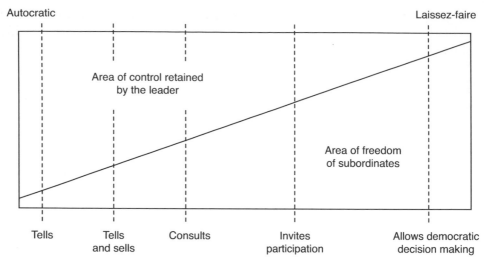

FIGURE 4.2 A continuum of leadership styles

Choice of leadership style is dependent not only on the situation but also on the maturity of the group. So to review those styles, we can now say the following.

○ **A telling style** is suited to an immature group which needs high levels of guidance and structure to get the task done and is less in need of relationship building. It can also be the only way to lead in a crisis when the outcome might be life-threatening. For example, when leading a team dealing with a cardiac arrest there is little time or opportunity to debate alternative courses of action. This should not mean, however, that the leader in such a situation should not be willing to check from time to time with colleagues in their team and listen carefully to ensure he or she is not missing anything critical.

○ **A selling style** emphasises both relationship and task behaviours and is suited to groups which are growing in maturity and are in need of support through a team-building process, but need to be regularly reminded of task direction. An example is if you decide you would like to arrange a mess dinner or medical school year reunion, and set out to persuade colleagues of the attractiveness of your idea.

○ **A consulting style** allows the leader to maintain a degree of control while permitting team members to influence practice and procedures. By listening to suggestions from team members the leader can often arrive at better decisions.

○ **A participating style** emphasises two-way communication and support but allows freedom to the team to make decisions which influence outcomes. This can create a sense of achievement and commitment to the task but it generally depends on team members being well trained and having a good understanding of team objectives. A decision to undertake a group or departmental audit project, for example, would require co-operation from all group members. Involving everyone in the decision would be most likely to achieve this.

○ **Delegating** can be used only with a mature well-trained team which is capable of managing its own tasks and relationships. The leader's role is more 'hands off', but still has accountability for results. This might include enlisting the help of more junior medical trainees, nurses or colleagues to manage an influx of work for which you are responsible.

Transformational leadership

We all have a preferred style to which we tend to revert when under pressure, but how can our leadership qualities and skills be developed? Assuming that the views outlined above are valid, it is *how you deal with people*, rather than *what you are* that makes the difference. Current thinking on leadership emphasises the role of the leader as one who influences, generates change and develops confidence in followers to take on responsibility for their own work outcomes.

This approach has come to be known as transformational leadership. Such leaders appeal to higher motives in their followers and focus on positive values when discussing team objectives. They work from a vision of the future rather than dependence on the past. Transformational leaders commit people to action, convert followers into leaders and convert leaders into agents of change. It might be helpful here to consider 'heroic' leadership. We tend to have developed our ideas of leadership from our own early life experience. This is likely to include reading novels and watching films or television programmes in which heroic figures lead from the front and always seem to be able to find the right solution to their followers' problems.

Transformational leadership does not sit comfortably with leadership as a 'heroic' process. Heroic leaders assume they should be at the heart of any important activity in which the team is involved. Heroic leaders are relied on by team members to know all the right answers, be aware of all that is going on in their area of responsibility and be capable of solving problems single-handed. They act as central decision makers and are regarded as being the only people who have the 'big picture'. These assumptions are seldom capable of being fulfilled in the complex world of modern organisations, although this does not stop some leaders from trying. Effective *post-heroic* leaders, including transformational leaders, share responsibility and challenge attempts to depend on them for all difficult decisions. They enable team members to achieve their own successes through coaching, support and personal development.

Psychodynamic approach

The psychodynamic approach to leadership developed during the 1960s and brought a humanistic perspective back into the work environment. This approach proposed that leadership style is influenced by family background and psychological make-up. It emphasised that effective leaders and followers are self-reflective and understand their personal preferences and those of the people around them. This recognises that effective leaders and followers have qualities and needs in common. The psychodynamic approach continues to have a wide-reaching influence on contemporary leadership theory and has contributed some of the field's most powerful tools, including the Myers-Briggs Type Indicator (*see* Chapter 1).

Organisational change

Change is normal in most contemporary organisations. The NHS is no exception. Change can sometimes feel as if it is imposed before there has been time to embed the last initiative. Medical professionals are generally cautious about change unless there is well-established evidence to support it. While this may be a sensible approach for treatments and procedures, it seldom applies to organisational change, which may be driven by economic necessity or by social or political circumstances.

There are generally held to be three steps in leading organisational change.

1 Recognition of the need for change. Effective leaders transmit this awareness to colleagues and followers and thus seek to create willingness for change.

2 The communication of a new vision which encompasses the long- and short-term needs of the organisation. A critical aspect of leadership is the ability to communicate effectively the benefits of the change to those most affected by it. Avoiding quick-fix solutions is critical to success, and this usually means a period of consultation with colleagues who may be able to refine the process.

3 The leader institutionalises the change by establishing new cultures and procedures and restructuring communication arrangements.

NHS Leadership Qualities Framework

The NHS Leadership Qualities Framework was developed from research into effective NHS leaders. It proposes 15 separate qualities in three clusters that are exhibited by successful leaders. These are as follows.

Personal qualities
These include:
○ self-belief
○ self-awareness
○ self-management
○ drive for improvement
○ personal integrity.

Setting direction
These include:
○ seizing the future
○ intellectual flexibility
○ broad scanning
○ political astuteness
○ drive for results.

Delivering the service
These include:
○ leading change through people
○ holding to account
○ empowering others

o effective and strategic influencing

o collaborative working.

This model provides the basis for developing leaders by its use as a 360-degree feed-back tool. You can find more information on each quality and its definitions at the Leadership Qualities Framework website (www.nhsleadershipqualities.nhs.uk).

Emotional intelligence

Leaders depend heavily on their ability to influence others. As we have seen, different styles of leadership may be suited to different situations. However, the most effective transformational leaders need to be self-aware and aware of the impact they have on others and to be able to work with this knowledge. Goleman (2000) argues that many aspects of our lives, including our impact as leaders, are dependent not on conventionally measured intelligence (such as Intelligence Quotient or IQ) but on a range of characteristics which have come to be called emotional intelligence, often referred to as EQ. In reviewing research into factors which led to success in life, Goleman reflected that academic intelligence offered virtually no preparation for the turmoil or opportunity brought by life's vicissitudes.

Emotional intelligence is said to comprise a set of capabilities. These are as follows.

Self-awareness

People with high self-awareness are able to identify their own emotions and the impact these have on their behaviour. They have a clear awareness of their own values and goals. They are also aware of their own strengths and weaknesses and are open to, and take heed of, constructive feedback about themselves. Their resulting self-assurance helps them to have an impact on others.

Self-regulation

People with this capability are good at managing their impulsive feelings and distress-ing emotions. They can think clearly under pressure. They are inclined to act ethically and maintain their high standards of behaviour. They normally work hard to meet commitments and to keep promises.

Self-motivation

Such people are results-oriented and strive to meet their objectives and standards. They align themselves with the goals of their team or organisation and are likely to make personal or team sacrifices for the benefit of the whole organisation. They persist in the face of opposition operating with the hope of success rather than fear of failure.

Social awareness

Those with this capability are sensitive to others' perspectives, attentive to emotional cues and good at listening. They are good at anticipating, recognising and meeting the needs of others with whom they interact closely, such as colleagues and patients. They tend to acknowledge and reward people's strengths and willingly act to develop others. They are good at recognising key power relationships and social networks and this makes them effective in the political arena.

Social skills

People with this capability are skilled at persuasion and can use complex strategies such as indirect influence to build consensus and support. They listen well and are effective in dealing with group issues in a straightforward manner. They lead by communicating their vision and engaging others in achieving it. They are good at identifying the causes of conflict and at negotiating and resolving disputes. They promote a friendly, co-operative climate while being prepared to encourage debate and open discussion.

The GMC Guidelines emphasise the importance of doctors' relationships with colleagues and patients. They also recognise the leadership role of consultants. Developing an emotional intelligence capability is a key part of medical training and such development continues throughout our working lives.

Getting results through others

Understanding what motivates people to achieve good results

Performance for anyone at work is generally dependent on three variables: their *ability*, which is a combination of aptitude and development; equipment and facilities must be available so they have the *opportunity*; and they must be *motivated*. In effect, performance is the product of ability and motivation.

Good leaders understand what motivates people and act to get the best from them. They must also harness those energies towards the successful achievement of goals. Motivation (in this context) is concerned with why people choose a particular course of action and persist in that action in preference to others. The underlying concept of motivation is the existence of *needs* which give rise to *drive* and *action* in order to achieve desired *goals* – thus meeting these needs and creating *satisfaction*.

Maslow's hierarchy of needs

Human needs were said by Maslow (1943) to be arranged in a hierarchy with basic needs dominating higher order needs until the former are reduced. His model is often presented as in Figure 4.3.

Physiological needs include food, water and warmth – the basic requirements of survival. Safety and security needs are met through freedom from threat of physical attack, protection from deprivation and by predictability and orderliness. Social needs are met by a sense of belonging, friendships and the giving and receiving of love. *Esteem* is focused on the self and involves the desire for confidence, status and the respect of others. Self-fulfilment (described by Maslow as self-actualisation) is the realisation of one's full potential. This may vary widely from one individual to another. Some authors have suggested that a sixth need which follows self-fulfilment is self-awareness.

Maslow argues that these needs are hierarchical, and that a need which is satisfied is no longer a motivator. Hence as lower-level needs are met so the driving force of behaviour becomes the higher need. Needs do not have to be fully met. There is a

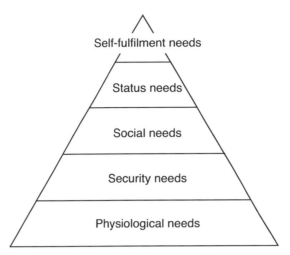

FIGURE 4.3 Maslow's hierarchy of needs

gradual emergence of a higher-level need as lower-level ones become more satisfied. He also makes it clear that the hierarchy applies to most, but not all, people. It is not necessarily a fixed order. Exceptions will be evident. Some people driven by a creative and self-actualising urge will ignore more basic needs. Others with high ideals or values may become martyrs and give up everything for the sake of their beliefs. It follows that in order to provide motivation for changes in behaviour a leader must direct attention to the next higher level of need.

Maslow's theory is difficult to test empirically. Those attempts which have been made give only tentative support. The theory has been influential nonetheless, perhaps because of its simplicity and universality.

McClelland's theory of motivation

The work of McClelland in 1976 led to a further content theory of motivation. He and his colleagues identified three main arousal-based, socially developed motive forces. These were: affiliation, power and achievement. These correspond broadly to Maslow's highest-order needs for love and society, esteem and self-actualisation. Their relative impact on behaviour varies with individuals as he has further asserted that although all of us possess all three needs we possess them in varying degrees; one person's highest-priority need may be achievement, whereas another person's may be affiliation or power. It was also possible to identify differences according to occupation.

Follow-up research focused on individuals with a high need for achievement in whom McClelland identified three common characteristics. You may recognise them in some of your colleagues:

o   a preference for personal responsibility
o   the setting of achievable goals
o   the desire for solid feedback on performance.

They like to be personally responsible for solving problems and getting results. They also like to attain success through their own efforts rather than as a member of a team. The recognition of others is not as important as their own sense of accomplishment. A second characteristic is the tendency to set moderate achievement goals and to take calculated risks. If the task is too difficult or too risky, the chances of success would be reduced. If the task is too easy or too safe, there would be little sense of achievement from success. Thirdly, feedback on performance should be prompt, clear and unambiguous. It helps to confirm success and give the sense of satisfaction which comes with achievement.

Herzberg's two-factor theory

Frederick Herzberg (1983) is among the best-known writers on motivation and has been influential in developing leadership thinking in relation to job content and the work environment and the impact on a person's commitment to work. His research indicated that job satisfaction and dissatisfaction at work nearly always arose from different factors and were not simply opposing reactions to the same. Herzberg wrote that the factors which motivate people at work are different to, and not simply the opposite of, the factors which cause dissatisfaction: 'Job satisfiers deal with the factors involved in doing the job, whereas job dissatisfiers deal with the factors which define the job context' (1959).

Thus, people who are dissatisfied with the context of their work (external factors to the job itself) will not normally be motivated by the job content. On the other hand, being satisfied with their context and environment is not motivational.

According to Herzberg, people have two sets of needs: one as an animal to avoid pain; and two as a human being to grow psychologically. Herzberg's 'two-factor' theory proposes that people at work can be dissatisfied by such factors as: working conditions, organisational policy, their status, security and salary. He described these as *'hygiene, or maintenance, factors'*. On the other hand, people express satisfaction when work provides them with a sense of achievement, recognition, advancement and responsibility. These are the *'motivators'*. Thus in order for leaders to motivate their team they must first ensure that the hygiene factors are correct. Only then can they hope to motivate them by providing them with work which allows a sense of achievement, recognition and responsibility.

In presenting evidence that salary did not motivate (it was more likely to cause dissatisfaction if it was considered inadequate or wrong), Herzberg argued that financial incentives which were used to increase effort soon became regarded by the worker as a right and ceased to have any motivational effect. There has been much debate about this view. However, Herzberg continued to argue his case for money as a hygiene factor – it must be seen to be fair but will not, of itself, increase output.

At the heart of Herzberg's theory is the need to provide people with work which can create a sense of satisfaction. This it will only do if the surrounding external factors are perceived to be acceptable to the worker.

Process theories

A second 'family' of motivational theories emphasises the study of process rather than content. These seek to provide a better understanding of the relationship between variables that influence work behaviour. Process models are generally more able to accommodate individual differences. Among the best known is '**expectancy theory**'. It emphasises an individual's perception of the probability that particular outcomes will result from specific courses of action. The model which is best known is based on three variables: *valence*, *instrumentality* and *expectancy*.

- **Valence** is defined as the attractiveness of, or preference for, a particular outcome to an individual. If a person has a preference for a particular outcome, valence is positive. Where avoidance of a particular outcome is preferred, valence is negative. If the person is indifferent to the outcome, valence is zero. Valence is the *expected satisfaction* and is distinguished from the value attached to the actual outcome once achieved.

- **Instrumentality** is best understood if we distinguish between first-level outcomes and second-level outcomes. First-level outcomes refer to actual performance in the work. For some, this will be an end to be valued for its own sake, as 'a job well done'. For others, the valence of the performance outcomes is determined by the second-level outcomes which may, for example, be derived from the financial gains resulting from satisfactory completion of the task. Second-level outcomes are need-related. Instrumentality is the extent to which first-level outcomes lead to second-level outcomes.

- **Expectancy** is a perception of the probability that the choice of a particular action will lead to the desired outcome. It relates effort expended to the achievement of first-level outcomes. This model, as with others derived from it, is useful in explaining the process by which people weigh and evaluate the attractiveness of different alternatives before committing themselves to specific courses of action. The models do not, however, reflect the actual decision-making steps taken by an individual.

Goal setting

Studies of goal-oriented behaviour provide a further insight into motivation. Goal setting may be viewed as a motivational technique rather than a theory. A number of organisational systems (such as performance appraisal) emphasise the importance of agreeing work goals with employees whose behaviour is thought to be determined by their goals. People's values give rise to emotions and desires which they strive to satisfy through their responses and actions. Goals direct work behaviour and performance and lead to certain consequences or feedback. People with specific measurable goals will perform better than those without. Also, those with difficult though achievable goals will perform better than those whose goals may be easily achieved.

In general, theories and models of motivation are unable to provide universal solutions to the challenge of motivating people at work. They do, however, help us to understand the complexity of the process and take us away from leadership approaches linked to fear and punishment once common among traditional managers earlier in the 20th century.

Developing team spirit

There are many kinds of team, some permanent, such as committees, some temporary, such as task forces and working groups. A good example of teamwork is the surgical team, which includes the surgeon and anaesthetist with juniors, nurses, operating department practitioners (ODPs) and others. Each is specialised and knows that each individual's success is dependent on the work of other team members. Bringing together the right number of people to work together does not necessarily make an effective team, as this takes time.

Team building and developing team spirit

Initially, there may be confusion over members' roles and leadership. Although there may be a nominal leader, others can contribute leadership roles at different times. Gradually, members identify their roles but sometimes as individuals working together rather than as a team. Conflicts and interactions occur as personal ideas and agendas are sorted. Gradually, the group comes to see itself no longer as a collection of individuals but as a group that has its own identity. There may even be experimentation with new roles. The group usually dies when the task has been completed. If the task changes, some members leave and others join. So the cycle continues and it is important to be aware of the dynamics of group behaviour.

Stages in team development

There are said to be four stages in the development of a team. Obviously, it is seldom this simple if individuals leave and others join. This also disrupts the process of team building. Some teams may never develop into a mature team. This may be due to a variety of reasons, depending on the mix of personalities within the team or the transient nature of the work. There is no particular timing to the stages – although they may be accelerated if attention is paid to helping the team through the stages of growth. The four stages are as follows.

1 **Forming:** this is the early, testing stage, with members being polite, watchful and guarded. Members try to learn about each other and may begin to project their personality through giving formal information about themselves.
2 **Storming:** there may be some confusion in the team, particularly about roles, with controlled conflict and confrontation, some opting out and difficulties may be experienced in agreeing tasks and goals.
3 **Norming:** the team starts to get organised and develop its skills, establish roles and procedures, giving feedback and confronting issues which are perceived to affect performance.
4 **Performing:** eventually, the team may mature to be resourceful, flexible, effective and supportive.

Some writers have added a fifth stage, which is sometimes called *adjourning* – that is to say that the team reaches a natural stage in its life when the demands made on it change to such an extent that it no longer needs to function as a team and so ends its life. Others describe this as the *mourning* stage – the implication here is that the team members become attached to the team to such an extent that personal grief affects team members at the natural end of the team's life.

Team maturity

The characteristics of a fully mature team are as follows.

- Team goals are clear and agreed.
- Information flows freely between members.
- Relationships between members are supportive, trusting and respectful.
- Conflict is regarded as natural and helpful, but it is on issues, not persons.
- The atmosphere is participative, open, non-threatening and non-competitive.
- Decisions are by consensus, although the team concedes to individual members the authority to make decisions when it would be most helpful to do so.

Remember it does not follow that because a group of people works together for sufficient time it will inevitably develop into a mature team. Nor is there a single approach to team building which is likely to work for all teams. One view is that the right mixture of personalities to make an effective team needs to be brought together in the first place. This, of course, is not usually possible since hospital teams are usually decided by the availability of staff at the time the team is formed.

Team maturity has implications for leaders. A recently formed team will require a higher level of direction in order to function. The leader's energies will be mostly taken up with making sure that individuals are clear about their roles, functions and goals. As the team develops and begins to be more focused on goal achievement, issues that arise around relationships will become evident and the team leader will find they are more engaged in supporting individuals and helping members to develop mutual understanding.

This relates to the storming stage, when the role of the leader is critical to ensuring the team continues to develop. Once the team members are sufficiently clear about team roles and their individual functions the leader will normally focus on building strong relationships within the team. Once this is established the mature team can be given increased responsibility for determining its own approaches and dealing with its conflicts (which are inevitable and normally healthy) in an effective manner without too much intervention from the leader.

Team roles

Research into teams by Meredith Belbin (2003) indicates that there are a number of separate team roles which, if working together, have a positive impact on team performance. These are often cited in team-development programmes. Belbin suggests the following roles are needed.

- **Plant:** concerned with putting forward ideas and strategies for achieving the objectives adopted by the group. Performance of this role requires creativity, imagination and innovation.
- **Resource investigator:** explores the environment outside the group by identifying ideas, information and resources. Performance of this role involves developing

contacts and co-ordination and negotiation with other groups and individuals.

○ **Co-ordinator:** organises, co-ordinates and controls the activities of the group. This involves the clarification of group objectives and problems, assigning tasks and responsibilities and encouraging group members to get involved in achieving objectives and goals.

○ **Shaper:** challenges, argues and disagrees. Usually, an achievement-motivated extrovert who has a low frustration threshold. He or she is a non-chairperson leader.

○ **Monitor evaluator:** involved in analysing ideas and proposals being considered by the team to evaluate their feasibility and value for achieving the group's objectives. It is important for the monitor evaluator to point out in a constructive manner the weaknesses of proposals being considered.

○ **Team worker:** creates and maintains team spirit. This involves improving communication by providing personal support and warmth to group members and by overcoming tension and conflict.

○ **Implementer:** is concerned with the practical translation and application of concepts and plans developed by the group. This entails a down-to-earth outlook coupled with perseverance in the face of difficulties.

○ **Completer finisher:** ensures that the group's efforts achieve appropriate standards and that mistakes of both commission and omission are avoided. It also involves searching for detailed mistakes and maintaining a sense of urgency within the group.

○ **Specialist:** is a key provider of the skills on which the team's particular output or service is based. They command the support of the team because of their knowledge, plus their dedication and pride in professional standards related to their particular skills and depth of experience.

More than one of these roles may be performed by a single person and it can assist team development if individuals can become aware of their preferred roles and work on these for the benefit of the team. Perhaps the most helpful thing to remember is that teams do not naturally fall into maturity – they need help, either from informed insiders or from someone who understands the mechanics of team building and can facilitate the process. If you feel the need for more practical advice, you therefore need to read the other parts of this section that are all relevant to successful team building.

Dealing with opposition: acting assertively

Assertion is not the same as aggression. Assertiveness has been defined as a quality demonstrated by individuals who know what they feel and what they want, take definite and clear action to express their views, refuse to be sidetracked and ensure others know where they stand. They do not try to serve their own interests at the expense of others. They are prepared to accommodate the interests of other people while not conceding more than they believe reasonable. Being assertive should usually result in both parties being satisfied with the outcome of the interaction.

○ An *aggressive* person seeks dominance, and aggressiveness involves attempts to intimidate others and violate their rights.

○ An *assertive* person exercises a right to express a viewpoint and have it fully heard, while respecting the rights of others.

A characteristic of clinical work is fragmentation and fluctuation in work rate. An essential skill needed by doctors in the protection of their work routines is the ability to prevent unnecessary disruptive interference. This is a common cause of frustration and impairs performance, particularly for those who hold supervisory responsibilities no matter how small. Working in teams means you need to be able to manage your work with others. Maintaining good working relationships while avoiding exploitation of goodwill can be difficult. Achieving and maintaining a satisfactory level of independence while still contributing fully to co-operative tasks requires a high level of social and group-working skills. Among these is the ability to act assertively when required − to decline taking on further demands when already fully loaded.

Responding to demands

There are many reasons why you may find it hard to say 'No' even to unreasonable demands that are made of you. The more obvious reasons are around the difficulty of deciding what tasks should, or should not, be a part of your role. Equally, you may be unable to define what a reasonable workload is. Job descriptions can help, but they are seldom sufficiently detailed to remove all uncertainty and, in any case, constant changes in detail mean they are seldom kept up to date.

It is difficult to deal with colleagues so that good relationships are always maintained without constantly succumbing to their demands. Unhealthy conflict can arise if we appear to be negative in our responses. It is suggested that in addition to 'fight or flight' responses to conflict, we have been conditioned to respond passively by parents who taught us to 'turn the other cheek'. Harris (1970) describes the impact of early life experiences on our later behaviours. In developing the concept of *transactional analysis* he outlines the nature of 'life scripts'. These are responses which we learn early in life and which help to shape our view of ourselves and hence our behaviour when responding to others.

Harris suggests that our behaviour is shaped by our use of life data which are derived from early experience of key relationships. Hence, interactions with others are shaped by our tendency to respond from the 'parent', 'adult' or 'child' within us. Since the interaction is two-sided, the type of initial message we receive frequently draws out the response we give. Parental instructions which are likely to be judgemental and directive tend to bring out the child in us, and vice versa. Overriding the tendency to behave in this predetermined manner is difficult. It requires the learning of new ways of reacting to requests and demands on our time.

Recognising 'assertive' rights

The first and most basic requirement we have in developing the ability to act assertively is to recognise the 'assertive rights' of human beings. Here are a few of them:

○ to judge your own behaviour, thoughts and emotions, and to take responsibility for their initiation and consequences upon yourself
○ to offer no reasons or excuses to justify your behaviour
○ to make mistakes – and be responsible for them
○ to be treated with respect as an intelligent, capable and equal human being
○ to express your feelings.

Assertive behaviour is not aggressive, nor is it passive. It does not infringe the assertive rights of others. It allows each party to depart with their own self-respect intact. Ideally, it should leave each party feeling 'OK'. It is usually concerned with helping individuals to acquire what is rightfully theirs and to say 'No' to what they do not want, or enable them to handle criticism.

Most people recognise their own need to behave assertively when they reflect on their inability to refuse requests for assistance from colleagues, friends or family members who they realise place unreasonable demands on their time or other resources. The early life conditioning referred to above is the most common reason for this weakness. Having convinced ourselves that we have a right to say 'No', the next task is to learn how to say it assertively.

Saying 'No'

There are two sides to saying 'No'. The first is to recognise how simple it is to find the word. It helps to practise saying it without apologising excessively or making complicated excuses. The dominant reason for experiencing difficulty in refusing an invitation or request is the feeling of guilt that results. The rights referred to above will, if remembered, help to assuage the guilt. As will the continued use of the skill so that it feels normal. A refusal to a request is not a rejection of the person making the request. Once this fact has been learned the process will become much easier to use. The other option is to develop the skill of refusal by using a tone which is friendly but firm. The way in which we look and express ourselves has a greater impact on the communication than the words we use.

Sometimes the person with whom we are dealing is persistent in their demands. This increases the challenge but need not create a problem. The key to success is calm repetition. This is sometimes referred to as the 'broken record'. It enables you to feel comfortable in avoiding manipulative verbal side-traps, argumentative baiting and irrelevant logic. Simply repeat your requirement or refusal in a calm and assertive manner until the other person accepts it.

Handling criticism

Handling manipulative criticism can cause difficulty. Assertive responses encompass a range of options. The first is to calmly acknowledge to the critic that there may be some truth in the criticism, yet leave yourself with the right to determine what you will do about it. A stage beyond this is to strongly agree with hostile or constructive criticism as it is given and accept your faults without resorting to denial. This has the effect of reducing your critic's anger or hostility without making you feel anxious or defensive. There is still no need to apologise if you do not wish to do so.

If it does not weaken your position, or threaten your self-respect, it is acceptable to seek a workable compromise with the other person. This involves recognising that a 'win–win' situation can be achieved by agreeing to concede something of your own position while retaining your right to protect your own needs.

The objective of assertive behaviour is not to win all your conflicts at the expense of someone else. Instead it is to maintain your own position and protect your rights as a person while dealing effectively with the demands of others around you. It should always be your aim to respect the equivalent rights of others. It is this which differentiates assertive from aggressive behaviour.

Guidelines for acting assertively

Skills of assertion can be identified and learned, increasing the ability to make a positive impact on others, a key factor for those in leadership roles. So let us consider some guidelines for exercising assertion in the face of the opposition!

o Build your argument step by step, thus ensuring people have the opportunity to understand your position.
o Say what you need from others because people need to know how they fit into larger plans.
o Communicate in language that others understand and feel makes sense.
o Avoid confused emotions; if you are angry, hurt or emotionally upset, others are more likely to respond to your feelings rather than your message. This can confuse the issues.
o Make it simple; people often lose the strength of their argument by excessive complexity or by dealing with several issues at once.
o Work towards resolving questions and concerns of others, which may involve continuing to put your message across until you are satisfied that a resolution can be achieved.
o Do not put yourself down; if something is important to you let others know where you stand.
o Watch out for 'flak'; others may try to divert you from your message. You may feel under pressure. Acknowledge their views but always return to your position.
o Error does not weaken; we all make mistakes and error should not make you feel inadequate. A sense of inadequacy will undermine your position.

People who face conflict assertively are said to:
o be open about their objectives
o establish what the other person's objectives are
o search for common ground
o state their case clearly
o understand the other person's case
o produce ideas to solve the differences
o build on and add to the other person's ideas
o summarise to check understanding and agreement.

Resolving conflict in work groups

Research prior to the first edition of this book confirmed the importance doctors attach to the effective working of the teams to which they belong. Occasionally, there can be tension and conflict in the team. This section helps to identify your approach to the handling of conflict. It does not relate to the conflict that can arise when patients complain, a subject dealt with in some detail in Chapter 6.

What is your preferred style when faced with conflict?

Conflict style inventory

This inventory is derived from Pfeiffer and Goodstein (1982. Choose a single frame of reference for answering all 15 items (e.g. work-related conflicts, family conflicts or social conflicts) and keep that frame of reference in mind when answering all items.

Allocate 10 points among the four alternative answers given for each of the 15 items below. For example: **'When the people I organise become involved in a personal conflict, I would usually ...'**

intervene to settle the dispute.	call a meeting to talk over the problem.	offer to help if I can.	ignore the problem.
3	6	1	0

Make sure your answers always add up to 10.

1 **When someone I care about is actively hostile towards me, i.e. threatening, shouting, abusive, etc., I tend to ...**

respond in a hostile manner.	try to persuade the person to give up his or her actively hostile behaviour.	stay and listen as long as possible.	walk away.

2 **When someone who is relatively unimportant to me is actively hostile toward me, i.e. shouting, threatening, abusive, etc I tend to ...**

respond in a hostile manner.	try to persuade the person to give up his or her actively hostile behaviour.	stay and listen as long as possible.	walk away.

3 When I observe people in conflicts in which anger, threats, hostility and strong opinions are present, I tend to . . .

become involved and take a position.	attempt to mediate.	observe to see what happens.	leave as quickly as possible.

4 When I perceive another person as meeting their needs at my expense, I am apt to . . .

work to do anything I can to change that person.	rely on persuasion and 'facts' when attempting to have that person change.	work hard at changing how I relate to that person.	accept the situation as it is.

5 When involved in an interpersonal dispute, my general pattern is to . . .

draw the other person into seeing the problem as I do.	examine the issues between us as logically as possible.	look hard for a workable compromise.	let time take its course and let the problem work itself out.

6 The quality that I value the most in dealing with conflict would be . . .

emotional strength and security.	intelligence.	love and openness.	patience.

7 Following a serious altercation with someone I care for deeply, I . . .

strongly desire to go back and settle things my way.	want to go back and work it out – whatever give and take is necessary.	worry about it a lot but not plan to initiate.	let it lie and not plan to initiate further contact.

8 When I see a serious conflict developing between two people I care about, I tend to . . .

express my disappointment that this had to happen.	attempt to persuade them to resolve their differences.	watch to see what develops.	leave the scene.

9 **When I see a serious conflict developing between two people who are relatively unimportant to me, I tend to . . .**

express my disappointment that this had to happen.	attempt to persuade them to resolve their differences.	watch to see what develops.	leave the scene.

10 **The feedback that I receive from most people about how I behave when faced with conflict and opposition indicates that I . . .**

try hard to get my own way.	try to work out differences co-operatively.	am easygoing and take a soft or conciliatory position.	usually avoid the conflict.

11 **When communicating with someone with whom I am having a serious conflict, I . . .**

try to overpower the other person with my speech.	talk a little bit more than I listen (feeding back words and feelings).	am an active listener (agreeing and apologising).	am a passive listener.

12 **When involved in an unpleasant conflict, I . . .**

use humour with the other party.	make an occasional quip or joke about the situation or the relationship.	relate humour only to myself.	suppress all attempts at humour.

13 **When someone does something that irritates me (e.g. smokes in a non-smoking area or jumps the queue in front of me), my tendency in communicating with the offending person is to . . .**

use strong direct language and tell the person to stop.	try to persuade the person to stop.	talk gently and tell the person what my feelings are.	say and do nothing.

14 When someone does something that irritates me (e.g. smokes in a non-smoking area or jumps the queue in front of me), my tendency in communicating with the offending person is to . . .

stand close and make physical contact.	use my hands and body to illustrate my points.	stand close to the person without touching him or her.	stand back and keep my hands to myself.

15 When someone does something that irritates me (e.g. smokes in a non-smoking area or jumps the queue in front of me), my tendency in communicating with the offending person is to . . .

insist that the person looks me in the eye.	look the person directly in the eye and maintain eye contact.	maintain intermittent eye contact.	avoid looking directly at the person.

Scoring and interpretation

When you have completed all 15 items, add your scores vertically, resulting in four column totals. Put these on the blanks below.

TOTALS =
Column 1 _____   Column 2 _____   Column 3 _____   Column 4 _____

o *Column 1– aggressive/confrontive:* High scores indicate a tendency to 'take the bull by the horns' and a strong need to control situations and/or people. Those who use this style are often directive and judgmental.
o *Column 2 – assertive/persuasive:* High scores indicate a tendency to stand up for oneself without being pushy, a proactive approach to conflict, and a willingness to collaborate. People who use this style depend heavily on their verbal skills.
o *Column 3 – observant/introspective:* High scores indicate a tendency to observe others and examine oneself analytically in response to conflict situations, as well as a need to adopt counselling and listening models of behaviour. Those who use this style are likely to be co-operative, even conciliatory.
o *Column 4 – avoiding/reactive:* High scores indicate a tendency toward passivity or withdrawal in conflict situations, and a need to avoid confrontation. Those who use this style are usually accepting and patient, often suppressing their strong feelings. Now total your scores for Columns 1 and 2 and Columns 3 and 4:

Column 1 + Column 2 = **Score A**
Column 3 + Column 4 = **Score B**

If Score A is significantly higher than Score B (25 points or more), it may indicate a tendency toward aggressive/assertive conflict management. A significantly higher B score signals a more conciliatory approach.

Conflict is certain to occur from time to time when people work closely together, especially if their work sometimes involves making difficult decisions together. Understanding how you normally react to conflict is the first stage in developing strategies for dealing with it in a way that suits your personality while achieving the best results in your own work. Colleagues respond differently according to a wide variety of factors, some of which might involve their current life pressures; others are more to do with their continuing view of themselves and others. Getting to know the things that are affecting other individuals can be as important as knowing yourself.

Handling conflict can and often does give rise to anger on either or both sides. We all feel anger sometimes and see it in others. But how can we personally handle our own and another person's anger?

Dealing with anger
Dealing with your own anger

Anger is a natural reaction, perhaps because of feelings that expectations were not met or somebody did or said something hurtful, and it can be destructive if not controlled. Generally, the earlier you tackle the cause the better, but it is likely to produce a better outcome if you can analyse the situation and decide what you are going to say to address the situation.

If you have been aggressive

You can be positive and direct but don't make it personal. Express your feelings – tell the other person how you felt but avoid saying the person made you angry. Perhaps acknowledge some responsibility for not saying something earlier but avoid putting yourself down, or becoming involved in retaliatory criticism or by airing past grievances. Don't stereotype, moralise or bring in third parties.

Apologising helps you become accountable for your own actions and may minimise anger and aggression in the future.

Remember to:
○ criticise the behaviour not the person
○ be specific and realistic in any request
○ avoid humour
○ use assertive language.

Some strategies for managing your own anger

If you have made your goal to be calm and effective here are some suggestions to try.
○ Review the kinds of situations that make you angry and look for a theme. Perhaps you feel your views are not being considered, maybe you feel threatened or feel you

are being treated unfairly? When avoidance is not an option we have to change how we view the situation.

- Consider your language; do you overreact to events? Was it a terrible thing that happened or was it merely irritating?
- Often people who become aggressive and angry fail to manage the situation. If you feel yourself becoming angry, get out of the situation diplomatically and take a break.
- Commit to being assertive instead of aggressive. Being assertive is standing up for yourself without hurting others. This sounds simple but it takes some effort to do when provoked. (*See* the section on assertiveness earlier in this chapter.)

Dealing with anger from someone else

Sometimes you will find yourself having to handle an angry colleague, a patient or patient's relative. Try to view anger in a rational way. The following points will help.

- Try to be on a level with the other person to avoid them feeling threatened.
- Keep your own voice as level as possible – try to communicate calmly.
- Allow them plenty of personal space.
- Acknowledge the other's feelings with an empathic statement. The other person may become aware that you understand their position.
- Indicate that you hear what is being said by reflective listening, repeating a summary of what you have heard.
- Avoid challenging an angry person.
- If you are in a closed space, check that you are well positioned for leaving quickly, or at least ensure that a large piece of furniture separates you from the complainant!

Use simple assertiveness techniques (*see* earlier in this chapter) such as the 'broken record' to express yourself calmly and persistently. An angry person often leaps from topic to topic.

(These points are more fully covered in Chapter 6 in the section on handling patients' complaints.)

Resources

- Mind, the mental health charity, has a booklet *How to . . . Deal with Anger*, available for downloads at www.mind.org.uk/assets/0000/0257/Howtodealwithanger2006.pdf.
- There are sources of information on anger management at NHS Choices at www.nhs.uk/conditions/anger-management/Pages/Introduction.aspx.
- And at NHS 24: www.nhs24.com/content/default.asp?page=s5_5&articleID=1890
- And at BUPA: hcd2.bupa.co.uk/fact_sheets/html/managing_anger.html.
- The Department of Health has material available at www.dh.gov.uk/en/Managingyourorganisation/Humanresourcesandtraining/NationalTaskForceonViolence/DH_4052018 but it is mainly devoted to the problem of violence against NHS staff. However, there is also an NHS website for conflict resolution.

Conflict resolution

Conflict is part of daily life, and arises from patients, relatives, colleagues and other NHS professionals including GP practices and even at home. Negative aspects of conflict are hard to manage. When our perception of a situation is negative perhaps because we lack resources, are tired, or have personal worries, we are less able to manage conflict effectively and we may become adversarial or angry. This may lead to defensive behaviour and taking criticism personally.

In April 2003 the NHS Security Management Service was established to ensure both its staff (and properties) became safe and secure. In addition to standardising security practices across the NHS, in April 2004 the Security Management Service devised a national syllabus for conflict resolution, which all employees who have contact with the public must complete (NHS Security Management Service, 2003, available as a pdf file at www.nhsbsa.nhs.uk/SecurityManagement/424.aspx). It provides a minimum standard for all frontline staff who have regular contact with the public either from meeting them face to face or via telephone calls. The module is applicable to NHS employees regardless of experience or specialty.

Delegation

Do you feel stressed and overloaded? There's only a limited amount that you can do, however hard you work. If you're good at your work, people will want to add to it and this can lead to pressure. You can't do everything that everyone wants as this can leave you stressed and unhappy. So you need to learn how to delegate. If you do this well, you can quickly build a strong and successful team. This is why delegation is such an important skill.

Delegation is not just about getting others to do the unpleasant, dirty, tedious or boring jobs that you do not want to do. It is also about sharing out the interesting things. You have a responsibility to help others, including junior colleagues, to develop and increase their experience. That will not happen unless you take steps to make it happen. You may not think this important now, but the more senior you become the more you will need to delegate. You can't do everything yourself. When you become a consultant you will have a great need to be skilful at delegation.

You may well feel that you have little need to consider the use of delegation skills, but as your career progresses you will need to learn. Some don't delegate because it takes a lot of effort. Time must be available for adequate training. Meaningfully involving other people develops those people's skills and abilities. This means that next time you can delegate with a high degree of confidence knowing the task will be done well with much less involvement from you. Delegation allows you to make the best use of your time and skills and it helps other people in the team grow and develop to reach their full potential.

Good time management involves making the most effective use of all staff resources, including your own. Tasks which can be carried out satisfactorily by others should not necessarily be routinely undertaken by you. The complex nature of healthcare demands specialist knowledge and skills. Rapid change brought on by technological development has increased the complexity of the work of doctors. It is impossible for an individual to carry all the knowledge and skills necessary to ensure effective performance of the unit. Delegation is not just about telling others to perform particular tasks. It provides a mechanism for controlled sharing of workload.

Delegation is achieving results by enabling and motivating others, usually those more junior to you, to carry out tasks for which you are ultimately accountable, to an accepted level of competence. The concept of delegation is simple. The practice is rather different and involves skill and understanding. Delegation is usually interpreted to mean passing down authority and responsibility to others at a more junior level. It is also possible to 'delegate laterally' to other specialist registrars and colleagues; for example, when a surgical specialist registrar hands over the responsibility for preparing a case for theatre, or when a medical specialist trainee hands over responsibility for a severe haematemesis to a surgeon. Even upward delegation may take place when, for example, a specialist trainee (ST) is called to an emergency elsewhere in the hospital the consultant may continue with the ward round or the theatre case that they were carrying out together.

Authority and responsibility

Authority and responsibility go together. Authority is the power and the right to take appropriate action in a given situation. Responsibility is an individual's 'answerability' for the successful accomplishment of a task. It would be unreasonable to delegate responsibility for an activity without giving the person authority to act. For example, if the ward phoned theatre to ask an anaesthetic specialist registrar for the analgesia of a previous case which had not been written up and a junior anaesthetic trainee was sent to write up the prescription, it would be unreasonable to expect the junior person to have to bring back the treatment sheet to be written up by the specialist registrar. Similarly, if a person is given authority, they should be held responsible for outcomes. If a trainee writes up the wrong dose or the wrong drug, the trainee is responsible for that error. This does not mean that a doctor can delegate *ultimate* responsibility. If the trainee was an FT1 and it was their first day, it might be considered unreasonable to delegate that task to them. The role is to delegate effectively and give support, encouragement and reasonable protection to staff. A doctor remains accountable for all the activities, whether medical or managerial, within his or her control.

Performance evaluation

Evaluation of performance and recognition of achievement are additional factors in the process of delegation. Effective control should mean that you would need to check on the satisfactory completion of the delegated task and give feedback.

Difficulties arise largely as a result of the emotional link we have with our own work. We worry that another person might not do it as well as we would or, worse, they might show us up by being much better at it! It is often easier to do it than explain to someone else how to do it. Sometimes we feel uncomfortable about asking others because they are too busy, or the task is unpleasant. There is the need to show trust in our juniors so that they can develop. A tension sometimes arises because of the nature of the 'trust/control relationship'. The amount of control we retain reduces with any increase in trust we demonstrate in the person to whom we delegate.

Motivation

I have already discussed what motivates people when we discussed leadership, but it might be useful just to repeat the key factors, as understanding how to motivate people is fundamental to success when delegating. Good leaders are able to understand what motivates their staff and act accordingly in order to get the best from them. The performance of any individual in the conduct of their work is likely to be dependent on three variables:

1 the *ability* to complete the task satisfactorily; this is a combination of aptitude and training
2 the equipment and facilities for the job must be available; they must have the *opportunity*
3 they must be *motivated* to complete the task.

Guidelines for successful delegation

Doctors work in teams that are made up of individuals who possess a complex range of skills and are often sensitive regarding their status in the team. Successful delegation requires careful thought and skill when dealing with individuals if good results are to be achieved.

Action

Identify a task that you perform and that you could ask a colleague or junior to do instead of you. It should be a task that you consider to be important, but not something that it would be unsafe to allow others less able to undertake.

- Identify a person to whom you could delegate the task. Take into account ability, personality and potential.
- Consult with the individual before finally deciding the extent of the delegated task.
- Delegate the *whole* task, not parts which do not carry significant responsibility.
- Clarify the purpose, limits and outcomes or expected results of the task.
- Provide them with relevant information and give clear guidance on what they should do if they need help.
- Be prepared to delegate enjoyable tasks as well as those which no one wants.
- Trust the person to get on with the task and allow them to decide when they need help, subject to agreed monitoring arrangements.
- Review their performance after a reasonable time has passed.
- Review your own performance. Note any improvement in the way in which you are able to carry out your core responsibilities.

The politics of influencing outcomes

Organisational relationships in hospitals are complex and involve most doctors in membership of a wide range of subgroups. Formal structures sometimes exist as diagrams showing divisions, directorates and so on, but these only partly describe the reality of groups or coalitions to which doctors (and others) relate or belong.

There are two broad categories of group – formal and informal. Sometimes informal groups, although not recognised in the formal structure of the hospital, have a very powerful influence on events.

One of the most valuable interpersonal skills is the ability to influence others. It can be used across hierarchical boundaries as well as in traditional managerial roles. Influence rests on the ability to use various forms of power. There are usually said to be five sources of power. Their suitability to exerting influence is affected by access to them and current circumstances. They are related to the following.

○ **Position** in the organisation: authority is vested in a post. This enables people in more senior positions to influence subordinates.
○ **Expertise** held by the post holder: others will usually defer to the person who (they perceive) has expert knowledge.
○ Control over **resources**: sometimes people have power well beyond their status in an organisation because they control access to resources that others need. Information might be regarded as a resource and control over information is sometimes used by relatively junior employees to exert influence over others.
○ Personal charm or **charisma**: there are a few people we meet who can influence others without appearing to have special powers other than their natural ability to lead. Some suggest these are simply people with unusually high levels of interpersonal skill.
○ **Coercion:** often exerted through an implied threat that induces fear in those who can be influenced by the possible outcome. Not regarded as an attractive option, it is sometimes used to achieve change in the face of opposition.

Another source of power is said to be **who you know** – this is a type of power gained by association or through access to information and influence not available to others. It can be useful but also carries a degree of risk if this is a major source of your influence, as it is largely outside your control.

Insight into the sources of power and those who control them can be a useful tool. Power and influence can sometimes be acquired by aligning with those who hold power. At other times it might be wise to avoid them.

Action

Write your name in the centre of a sheet of paper. Now write in the names and/or job titles of all those with whom you interact in your work and work-related activities, particularly those who may have more influence in your organisation than you. You can also add your social contacts.

Group these into formal contacts by drawing lines between connected names. Some names or titles are likely to be part of your *informal* network. Circle these and then list them separately.

Consider whether any of these are particularly influential in the context of the organisation. How could they help you to achieve your personal goals? How do you relate to them at present? Could you do more to employ their strengths on your own behalf?

What sources of power do you currently exploit?

Which others could you exploit?

Which do you encourage those working with or for you to develop?

Handling stress
Personality Types A and B

Personalities and their approach to work-related stress have been assessed according to type. Complete the following questionnaire. Answer each question 'yes' or 'no'.

- Do you characteristically do several things at once (e.g. telephoning, reading your post and jotting notes on a pad)?
- Do you feel guilty when relaxing as if there is something else you should be doing?
- Are you quickly bored when other people are talking? Do you find yourself wanting to interrupt or get them to hurry up?
- Do you try to steer conversation towards your own interests instead of wanting to hear about the interests of others?
- Are you usually anxious to finish each of your tasks so that you can get on to the next?
- Are you unobservant when it comes to anything that is not immediately connected with what you are actually doing?
- Do you prefer to have rather than to be (to experience your possessions rather than to experience yourself)?
- Do you do most things (eating, talking, walking) at high speed?
- Do you find people like yourself challenging and people who dawdle infuriating?
- Are you physically tense and assertive?
- Are you more interested in winning than in simply taking part and enjoying yourself?
- Do you find it hard to laugh at yourself?
- Do you find it hard to delegate?
- Do you find it almost impossible to attend meetings without speaking up?
- Do you prefer activity holidays to relaxing ones?
- Do you push those for whom you are responsible (children, subordinates, partner) to try to achieve your own standards without showing much interest in what they really want out of life?

It has been suggested that personality types can be divided into those who are driven by ambition and the need to achieve (Type A), and those more laid-back people for whom life is a series of experiences which may be outside their control but can be nonetheless enjoyable (Type B). People with extreme Type A personalities will have answered 'yes' to all 16 questions above.

If you have responded positively to 12 or more of the questions, you are likely to have significant Type A tendencies. Type A people like deadlines and pressures, are impatient to move on to new challenges and can be intolerant of the failure of others to measure up to their own standards of commitment. Unfortunately, this approach to life can lead to Type As drawing more upon themselves than they can reasonably cope with and finding they have fewer coping mechanisms as the pressure rises to breaking point.

If you scored 8 or less you are probably a Type B. The Type B personality is relaxed, uncompetitive and inclined to reflection and self-analysis.

How stressed are you?

Most of us can manage varying amounts of pressure without feeling stressed. In order to fully understand the stress in our lives, we need to assess the demands that are made on us and indeed we make on ourselves and our capacity for handling stress. People vary and what appears as a major problem to one person may be an exciting challenge to another.

Some may be suffering relationship problems, bullying, problems at home, some from the stress inherent in medicine. Doctors find it difficult to acknowledge stress, feeling that they should be able cope because they are doctors (Firth-Cozens and Morrison1989).

However, too much pressure can overstretch our ability to cope and then stress is experienced. Because everyone reacts to stress in different ways, no one stress test can give you a complete diagnosis of your stress levels, but the answers to the following questions may give some indication of your stress level. So let's try it.

I feel that:
- there aren't enough hours in the day to do everything I need to
- that there are too many deadlines to meet
- I bring work home
- I am spending longer and longer on the wards
- I ignore problems and hope that they will go away
- I don't perform tasks as well as I used to, my judgement is clouded and not so good
- I'm getting more and more disorganised
- I do jobs myself to ensure they are done properly
- I think about problems when I should be relaxing
- I tend to underestimate how long it takes to do things
- I have a tendency to eat, talk, walk and drive quickly
- I feel guilty about relaxing and doing nothing
- I feel tired when I wake up
- I finish other people's sentences for them when they speak slowly
- I'm too busy to eat, skipping meals or suffer loss of appetite or sometimes eat for comfort

- ○ I feel angry and irritated if the car or traffic in front seems to be going too slowly
- ○ I become very frustrated at having to wait in a queue
- ○ if something or someone really annoys me I bottle up my feelings
- ○ when I play sport or games, I always want to win
- ○ I have mood swings, difficulty making decisions, my concentration and memory is impaired
- ○ I find fault and criticise others rather than praising, even when deserved
- ○ when I listen, I am preoccupied with my own thoughts
- ○ I suffer with bruxism
- ○ I get aches and pains in the neck, head, lower back and shoulders
- ○ I have a dependency on alcohol, caffeine, nicotine or drugs
- ○ my self-confidence and self-esteem are lower than I would like them to be
- ○ my sex drive is lower/I experience changes to my menstrual cycle
- ○ I don't have time for many interests or hobbies outside of work.

Count up the number of positive responses that apply to you. If you have

- ○ 4 points or less it means you are least likely to suffer from stress-related illness.
- ○ 5–13 points suggests you are more likely to experience stress-related ill-health, either mental, physical or both and would benefit from stress management or advice to help in the identified areas.
- ○ 14 points or more, you are the most prone to stress. You might even be heading for some of the stress-related illnesses, physical or mental, maybe not now but in the future, and need to consider small practical changes to improve your life.

Action

Given that we all have pressures in our lives, all of which have the potential to cause worry and stress, construct a worksheet to identify the pressures, learn how to eliminate excessive worry and so increase well-being and potentially your health. List all of your current worries and their sources. Try to be as specific as you can by thinking about your whole life: work, commuting, home, family, relationships, communication issues, finances, organisational problems, changes to routine, health concerns, major life events, in fact anything that causes you to worry.

List worries and their sources in columns:

Worry	Source	Score

Now consider each separately and ask yourself, on a scale of 1–10, where 1 is only *slightly* worrying and 10 is *extremely* worrying, 'How important is this worry?' and score each one.

Now quickly re-enter them onto another sheet, putting it in one of the two columns depending on whether this is something you have 'some control' over or 'no control'. Those in the first column that you cannot control may as well be let go at least for the moment or at least defer them, so you might as well stop spending time on them. Just concentrate all your efforts on what you have put in the right-hand column, going through this list and prioritising each one in order of which ones are the most important to you in term of your stress levels right now.

Important worries I have some control over	Actions I can take to reduce this worry

Finally, from this list put the five most important worries that you do have an element of control over into a plan of action chart.

You must follow through and put these actions into effect, being realistic and not doing it all at once. Focus on what is most important even if it is just one thing. You may need to list what you need to make it happen. You may need to get someone to help and support you, but set yourself a realistic target and date to achieve a result. Commit yourself and get a real sense of achievement. You will then start to decrease your worry, feel calmer, more relaxed and less stressed!

Practical ways of handling stress

Learn to manage your time more effectively

Avoid wasting time with unimportant tasks when stressed. Learn to prioritise your day and do important jobs first. The unimportant ones can wait and will sometimes disappear. But don't put off all the unpleasant tasks as avoidance can cause more stress. It is often better to give unpleasant tasks a high priority and do them first. You might also want to read the section on time management later in this chapter.

Lifestyle

Maintaining a balanced lifestyle is seen as essential to healthy stress levels. This helps to ensure that workload does not go beyond an individual's capacity for managing the work, although this is easier said than done. It requires strict time management and measures to assist in coping with stress. Changing a lifestyle is not easy but can be managed and is better than the effects of failure to do so. Type A personalities, para-doxically, can be most effective in implementing change programmes. Finding and developing non-work interests that provide an antidote to overwork are a good start to the process. Competitive sports not only improve physical fitness but separate you from work pressure for significant periods of time. Learning to delegate (*see* earlier section in this chapter) is also vitally important for people with Type A personalities.

Know and accept your limitations and don't take on too much. We often increase our stress because we want to be liked and don't want to let people down, so we end up trying to do more than is practical. So learn to delegate effectively (*see* p. 132) and be more assertive (*see* earlier in this chapter on dealing with conflict and acting assertively) so that you can say no without offence.

Find out what causes you stress

Try to discover what is worrying you and attempt to change your thoughts and beha-viour to reduce it. A stress assessment (*see* earlier in this chapter 'How stressed are you?') might help you understand the causes and implications and assist in helping you manage, cope and make changes.

Avoid unnecessary conflict

Try not to be argumentative and ask yourself whether the conflict or argument is worth the stress. Look for win–win solutions and try to resolve a dispute where both parties feel there is some positive outcome. If necessary, find out the real cause of the problem.

Accept the things you cannot change

Changing a difficult situation is not always possible. If this proves to be the case, recognise and accept things as they are and concentrate on the things you have some control over. Managing change is an essential quality to develop.

Take time out to relax

Always make sure you take a holiday of at least 10–14 continuous days. Bear in mind that work is performed more effectively if you take short breaks during the day of 10–15 minutes. Time is made up easily by improvements in work rate.

Another relaxing break is to meet friends with whom you can engage in out-of-work activities that involve having fun. Stress is also helped by some form of physical activity (*see* 'Lifestyle' above).

Some writers on stress management advocate the use of relaxation and meditation techniques. These range from undertaking simple physical exercises to the acquisi-tion of understanding of Eastern philosophies and habits of mind. They do not work for everyone. Try them in case they are right for you. Certain personalities will feel unhappy with this type of approach and it requires practice to become competent so you should persevere before deciding it does not work for you. Perhaps try meditation or relaxation techniques for only five minutes the first few times, rising to 10 minutes or more after a week or so. This approach does not remove the sources of stress. In serious situations radical life change may be necessary, such as a change of career direction. Meditation and other techniques are, arguably, a way of managing stress rather than allowing it to manage us.

Develop a positive thinking style

Try to see the situation differently and talk it over with somebody before it gets out of proportion. Often just talking to a friend/colleague/family member will help you see things from a different perspective.

Avoid alcohol, nicotine and caffeine as coping mechanisms

Long term these coping mechanisms will just add to the problem. Caffeine and nicotine, being stimulants, may just increase stress and even cause anxiety. Although alcohol is a depressant, it is no answer. According to some authors some juniors are already flirting with alcohol and drug misuse. The need for help for stress in health professionals is now widely recognised (Firth-Cozens and Payne 1999; King *et al.* 1992; Scott *et al.* 1995).

It has also been suggested that the NHS could reduce stress in trainees by:

o good career advice
o removing unnecessary tasks from juniors
o good domestic arrangements while living in
o an effective and supportive appraisal and feedback system
o fixed teaching sessions for consultants within their contract
o a stress support service.

As far as the last item is concerned, some deaneries have already set up support services and networks and details of these should be available through your deanery website.

NHS as employer and stress: useful sites for information

Department of Health Work Related Stress policies (2007) are available to read at www.dh.gov.uk/en/Managingyourorganisation/Humanresourcesandtraining/Model employer/Occupationalhealth/DH_4063966. They set out the measures being taken to reduce stress and the causes of stress in the NHS and discuss the recognised causes of stress and Health and Safety legislation.

NHS Employers provide advice and guidance to NHS organisations on a wide range of healthy workplace issues including health and safety, mental health and stress, providing guidance on workplace stress with the following headings:

o stress management
o employers' responsibilities
o healthy lifestyles
o getting help
o campaign materials
o recognising stress
o benefits of tackling stress
o resources
o what employers should do

o management practices
o court cases and related stress.

The NHS Employers website to access these documents is at www.nhsemployers.org/
HealthyWorkplaces/Pages/Home-Healthy.aspx.

The NHS Choices website has information on symptoms, causes, diagnosis, treatment, complications and prevention of stress, together with the views of a stress expert
and other links; it is available at www.nhs.uk/conditions/stress/Pages/Introduction.
aspx?url=Pages/what-is-it.aspx.

Characteristics of those who handle stress well

Finally, the characteristics of those who handle stress well include the following.

o Shelving problems until they are capable of dealing with them.
o Relaxing after coping with demanding and stressful tasks, usually undertaking
  contrasting activities.
o Taking a wider view of situations and not becoming bogged down in detail.
o Controlling the build-up and pace of stressful situations by planning and inter-
  vening to prevent themselves from becoming swamped.
o They are prepared to confront difficulties or unpleasant issues.
o They know their own capacity and do not permit themselves to become overwhelmed by events.
o They can cope with being unpopular.
o They do not commit themselves to very tight deadlines which are unlikely to be
  met.
o They put limits on their involvement in work in order to maintain a balanced
  lifestyle.

The above section on stress management is intended to provide an insight into the
issues. It does not deal with the responsibility that those supervising the work of others
have in ensuring safe and realistic work programmes for them.

Making effective use of your time

Time is a remarkable commodity. No matter how we waste time today, tomorrow's
entitlement remains untouched. Most junior doctors recognise the problem of time
management. You need to organise your work around structured sessions and your
work makes multiple demands on your time. Then there is your private life and finding
time for family, friends – even for yourself! Few have found a simple solution. Most
do their best but some manage better than others. This is partly based on differing
personalities. Some people like their lives to be conducted with a high measure of order
and structure. Others prefer to keep their options open and not have plans that might
inhibit their flexibility, taking opportunities as they arise (Houghton 2004). Regardless
of our natural preferences, work imposes demands that, if not met by careful organisation and planning, can lead to stress and even failure.

If you master time management skills you'll find that you take control of your workload. At the heart of time management is an important shift in focus as people spend their days in a frenzy of activity achieving very little. This is because they're not concentrating their effort on the things that matter the most.

The 80:20 Rule

Summed up as the Pareto Principle, the '80:20 Rule' (Pareto 1971) says that typically 80% of unfocused effort generates only 20% of results, so 80% of results are achieved with only 20% of the effort. While the ratio is not always exactly 80:20 it is a broad but true generalisation. So by applying the time management efforts you could optimise your effort to ensure that you concentrate as much of your time and energy as possible on the high-payoff tasks to achieve the greatest benefit within limited time.

How good is your time management?

How well do you use your time? Try to answer the following as honestly as you can. Place a cross (X) in the appropriate column for each item and check your result using the scoring system underneath.

		Not at all	Rarely	Sometimes	Often	Very often
1	I work on highest priority tasks first.					
2	I never complete tasks at the last minute or have to ask for extra time.					
3	I carefully plan and schedule work.					
4	I know exactly how much time I'm spending on various jobs.					
5	I find my work tends to mount up; too much other paperwork and emails to deal with.					
6	I plan which tasks and activities to work on.					
7	I plan in contingency time to deal with anything unexpected.					
8	I know which tasks are high, medium or low value.					
9	When starting a new task I analyse it for importance and prioritise it accordingly.					
10	I am stressed about deadlines and commitments and never have time to just think.					
11	Distractions such as the phone often keep me from getting on with important tasks.					
12	I take work home to catch up as the only way to cope.					

	Not at all	*Rarely*	*Sometimes*	*Often*	*Very often*
13 I prioritise my 'to-do' list.					
14 I generally feel out of control in my career and life.					
15 Before I undertake a task I check that the result will be worth the time and effort put in.					

For statements 1, 2, 3, 4, 6, 7, 8, 9, 13 and 15 the columns score 1 to 5.

For statements 5, 10, 11, 12 and 14 the columns score 5 to 1.

○ If your score is 46–75 you're managing your time very effectively, but you could find something useful in the sections below in case you could tweak things to make your life even better.

○ From 31–45 you're good at some things with room for improvement elsewhere. Read the sections below and concentrate on the relevant issues and work may become less stressful.

○ And if your score is 15–30 the good news is that you've got an opportunity to improve your time management skills by reading below.

As you answered the questions, you probably had some insight into areas where your time management could be improved, so here is a quick review with suggestions for each skill required.

Goal setting (Statements 6, 10, 14, 15)

To manage time effectively you need to set goals in order to avoid frittering away your time. People tend to neglect goal setting because it requires time and effort but a little expended now saves an enormous amount of time, effort and frustration in the future. As a doctor you need to manage simultaneous tasks such as dealing with an emergency admission and managing another patient about whom you are concerned and who is located on a different ward. This is before you take account of your private life. The first thing to recognise is that, when thinking about organising your life, it is unhelpful to separate work and 'non-work'.

Take a sheet of paper and write down your 'foreseeable life goals'. These are likely to be attainable within the next two or three years. Think of them as starting from now. They might be personal, family, social, career, financial, community or spiritual. Work quickly without limiting your ambitions.

Next, review and refine these goals into statements that imply action. Some may be immediate – 'Spend more time with my family'. Defining and securing your career objectives are likely to figure large. Others may require considerable balancing of resources and long-term planning such as investing to secure early retirement. Some may be unrealistic and should be disregarded at this stage.

Prioritisation (Statements 1, 4, 8, 9, 13, 15)

Prioritise your list. This involves taking decisions about yourself. Prioritising what needs to be done is especially important. Without it you may work very hard but you won't be achieving the results you desire because what you are working on is not of strategic importance.

Most people often have a 'to-do' list. The problem is they are just a collection of things that need doing. The plan is unstructured. To-do lists can be top down, bottom up, easiest to hardest. To work efficiently you need to work on the most important, highest-value tasks. This way you won't get caught scrambling to get something critical done as the deadline approaches. It can be difficult but not as difficult as living without purpose. They will all be important but some will be more important than others. Use them to develop your approach to time management.

Interruptions (Statements 5, 9, 11, 12)

Having a plan and knowing how to prioritise it is one thing but you need to know how to minimise the interruptions to your priorities.

Procrastination (Statements 2, 10, 12)

'I'll do it later' is such an easy thing to say to yourself, but after too many such decisions the work piles so high that it seems insurmountable. It is often said that procrastinators work as many hours in the day as other people, often working longer hours but wasting time on the wrong tasks. Some of the possible causes are:

o   feeling overwhelmed by the task
o   not knowing where to begin
o   waiting for the 'right' mood or the 'right' time to start
o   underdeveloped decision-making skills
o   poor organisational skills
o   perfectionism – I don't have the skills/resources to do this perfectly so I won't do it yet.

Procrastination is appealing but fatal. The best way to overcome the temptation is to recognise the habit. Then you can decide why you do it. Once you know why, you can plan to overcome it, perhaps by rewarding yourself for getting jobs done and thinking regularly of the consequences of not getting on with things. And just a note to remember that putting off an unimportant task isn't procrastination; it's probably good prioritisation (*see* below).

Scheduling (Statements 3, 7, 12)

Essentially, time management comes down to planning the use of your time. When you have decided on priorities create a realistic schedule that will keep you on track and protect you from stress. Make sure you leave room for interruptions and contingency time for those unexpected events.

Develop a sense of time: how do you really spend your day?

Analyse your working day by keeping a time log for a few days. You can use an ordinary desk diary. Record the activity in which you are engaged at 15-minute intervals throughout the day. The first time you use an activity log you may be shocked to see the amount of wasted time!

List the activities and record the time spent on each in a typical week. Ask yourself if this reflects your priorities. Are there activities that take up time but contribute little or nothing? What would happen if you stopped doing them completely? How much of your time do you keep to use at your discretion? Some authors on time management also suggest that as well as recording activities, you should note how you feel, whether alert, flat, tired, energetic, etc. Do this periodically throughout the day. You may then decide to integrate your activity log with a stress diary.

Reviewing your log you may be alarmed to see the amount of time you spend doing low-value jobs. You may also see that you are energetic in some parts of the day and flat in others. Perhaps this depends on the rest breaks you take, the times you eat and the amount you eat, and the quality of your nutrition. The activity log gives you some basis for experimenting with these variables within the limitations set by your timetable. For example, freeing up extra time for the most challenging tasks when your energy is highest and restricting personal activities such as sending non-work emails to when you are less energetic.

Planning and prioritising

Write down all of the tasks that you need to do and if they are large break them down into their smaller components to make them manageable. You might want to use a sheet of paper, personal organiser, wall chart or desk diary. Allocate priorities into groups, say A (very important, or very urgent) to E or F (unimportant, or not at all urgent). If too many tasks have a high priority, run through the list again and demote the less important ones. Once you have done this rewrite the list in priority order.

Set aside time at the beginning of each day to list your tasks and prioritise them. Again you can use a system of letters or stars to indicate priority.

   ***   Must be done today.
   **   Should be done today.
   *   Might be done today.

It is crucial to understand the difference between tasks that are urgent and those that are important. Urgent but unimportant tasks could be delegated or done quickly but given a smaller amount of your time. Important but non-urgent tasks can be scheduled for later in the day, week or month and given sufficient space in your diary to complete them properly at the first sitting. Some tasks will be a mixture of both. One way of representing this is shown in Figure 4.4.

Work through your list, completing each task before moving on to the next. Set a time limit for each task based on its priority. As a doctor and specialist registrar some of your time will be largely outside your control. But it is not all out of your control. You will be surprised to find how much you can control if you choose. Use your daily

Urgent	Non-urgent
I Crises Pressing problems Deadline-driven problems	II Prevention Relationship building New opportunities Planning
III Interruptions Some calls, emails, letters Local pressing matters Popular activities	IV Trivia Some mail Some phone calls Gossip

FIGURE 4.4 Time management matrix

planning session to make best possible use of the time that you can influence. Do not worry if, at the end of the day, you have not completed all of your tasks. Simply delete those that are no longer necessary and transfer the rest to your list for the following day. Remember to allocate time to deal adequately with the demands of quadrant II – this is the way to reduce the number of tasks that find their way into quadrant I.

Working routines

Incoming paperwork should be handled only once. Never put a pathology or X-ray report down until you have decided what action to take, even if only to ask for advice. Do not put a letter or memo down until you have written or dictated a reply. If you really cannot act immediately, do something, even if it is just to put it on your to-do list and allocating it appropriate priority.

Writing clearly, simply and concisely is essential for effective first-time communication. Consider the purpose of your communication, jot down key points and then arrange them in a logical order. Use short sentences, avoiding jargon and formal language.

o Emails can be a time waster or a tremendous time saver particularly now that emails are available on your mobile phone. Read and respond to emails only at designated times during the day, for example at the beginning of the day, before lunch and again before you leave work. Remember that used appropriately, email is an excellent way to convey information. It can be more precise than voicemail. The sender and receiver have a record of the communication and more information can be conveyed and at a convenient time.

o Reading is an important method of personal development for doctors. Develop good habits when dealing with paperwork. Scan lengthy documents to decide whether you need to read them all. Perhaps read only the introduction and summary or conclusions for some. Highlight key points so that you can refer to them easily. 'Speed-reading' can be useful for those with many large documents to absorb but is no substitute for good judgement when deciding what to read!

❍ Telephones save time when used appropriately. Try keeping a time log of your telephone use during one week. You may be surprised at the total time taken up. Before using the telephone make a quick note of what you wish to say. Keep the conversation on track and bring it to a polite end when you have completed your business. Mobile phones can be a mixed blessing. Ask yourself: 'Does keeping it switched on give me more, or less, control over my life?'

❍ Avoid procrastination. When faced with large or difficult tasks most of us are inclined to find diversions in order to avoid starting. Set yourself a starting time for tasks you might be tempted to put off. Forget about finishing the task – concentrate on starting it. Make your deadlines public. Reward yourself for completing unpleasant tasks. Learn to say 'No' to unreasonable or low-priority requests from others. It takes practice to do this assertively and without offending.

Working with others

❍ Meetings can waste a lot of your time. Ask yourself if the meeting is necessary or if you even need to attend. If you have called the meeting, prepare an agenda, set a time limit and communicate these to others before it starts. Encourage them to prepare for the meeting. Discourage irrelevant discussion. There is a separate section on meetings in Chapter 3.

❍ Delegation can be painful. Giving away tasks you enjoy, or feel you cannot trust others to do, may be the only way to release time for what you need to do to achieve results. There is more on delegation earlier in this chapter.

❍ Saying 'No' to impossible or unnecessary tasks is often more difficult than it should be. We are brought up to acquiesce to our seniors rather than challenge them and this creates habits that are nearly impossible to break. Assertive behaviours are dealt with earlier in this chapter.

Shifts and handovers

The shift patterns of medicine now require doctors to make good handover of patient care essential. Shift work relies heavily on effective information transfer at handover to protect patient safety. Inadequate handover of clinical information carries significant risks for individual clinicians, their organisations and their patients. Many patients have suffered adverse consequences when a handover goes wrong (BMA 2004). Poor handover has the potential to precipitate error in an otherwise adequate management plan and cause harm to patients.

Key information is provided by the BMA brochure *Safe Handover: Safe Patients: guidance on clinical handover for clinicians and managers*, available online at: www.bma. org.uk/images/safehandover_tcm41–20983.pdf and endorsed by the GMC (GMC 2006), whose own guidelines regarding handover state that you must be satisfied that suitable arrangements are in place for patient care when staff you manage are off duty and that effective handover procedures are followed.

Essentially, it is about good communications. You can improve your own work schedule simply by taking a little time and trouble; for instance, taking trouble and care at handover.

Handover also requires organisation in a department, ensuring support and bringing together the relevant medical, nursing and non-medical personnel. It's an exercise that requires consultant involvement. They, in turn, will need the support and help of senior nurses and possibly managers. As a junior doctor your most important role in improving work schedules will be in selling the issue to your peers, particularly to your senior colleagues.

Some of the key features of effective handover are as follows.

○ It is a protected time with sufficient time for the handover and with an overlap between staff of 15–30 minutes to allow for adequate communication.
○ It should be pager bleep-free except for emergencies.
○ It takes place in working time.
○ There should be clear leadership by the most senior clinician present.
○ Information should be given about all patients, not just sick ones, enabling the new doctor to be in a position to judge easily any changes in a patient's condition.
○ It should give the accurate location of all patients.
○ Keeping written records of plans thus ensuring nothing important is forgotten due to pressure of new work.
○ Keeping your own daily written record.

For more detailed information read the BMA brochure mentioned above (*Safe Handover: Safe Patients*). There is also a useful booklet by the Australian Medical Association available at www.ama.com.au/system/files/node/4064/Clinical_Handover.pdf.

Action

Think back over the last fortnight.
● When starting on-call periods, have you always felt adequately briefed about the inpatients under your care?
● When coming on duty in the morning, when and how have you learnt about new patients admitted over the on-call period?
● When going off duty in the evening, have you and your colleagues always fully briefed the on-call team about your patients?

Related reading

Back K, Back K. *Assertiveness at Work*. Maidenhead: McGraw-Hill; 2005.

Belbin M. *Management Teams: why they succeed and fail*. London: Butterworth Heinemann; 2003.

BMA. *Safe Handover: Safe Patients: guidance on clinical handover for clinicians and managers*. BMA, NHS Modernisation Agency and NHS National Patient Safety Agency; 2004. Available online at: www.bma.org.uk/images/safehandover_tcm41–20983.pdf

Covey SR. *The Seven Habits of Highly Effective People*. London: Simon and Schuster; 2004.

Crainer S (ed). *Leaders on Leadership*. Corby: Institute of Management Foundation; 1996.

Darzi A. *Next Stage Review: high quality care for all, The Darzi Report 2008*. London: Department of Health; 2008. Available online at: www.dh.gov.uk/en/publicationsandstatistics/publications/publicationspolicyandguidance/DH_085825

Firth-Cozens J, Morrison LA. Sources of stress and ways of coping in junior house officers. *Stress Med*. 1989; **5**: 121–6.

Firth-Cozens J, Payne R. *Stress in Health Professionals*. London: Wiley; 1999.

Fontana D. *Managing Stress*. London: British Psychological Society/Routledge; 1989.

Gill R. *Theory and Practice of Leadership*. London: Sage Publications; 2006.

GMC. *Good Medical Practice*. London: General Medical Council; 2006.

Goleman D. *Working with Emotional Intelligence*. New York: Bantam; 2000.

Gourlay R. *Dealing with Difficult Staff in the NHS*. London: Kogan Page; 1998.

Harris TA. *I'm OK. You're OK*. London: Pan; 1970.

Herzberg F. *The Motivation to Work*. New York: John Wiley; 1959.

Herzberg F. One more time: how do you motivate employees? *Harvard Business Review*, 1987; **65**(5): 109–20.

Herzberg F, Mausner B, Snyderman BB. *Herzberg on Motivation*. Cleveland, OH: Penton/IPC; 1983.

Houghton A. Understanding personality type: introducing personality type. *BMJ Career Focus*. 2004: **328**: 177–8.

Howkins E, Thornton C. *Managing and Leading Innovation in Health Care: Six Steps to Effective Management Series*. London: Bailliere Tindall; 2002.

King MB, Cockroft A, Gooch C. Emotional distress, sources, effects and help sought. *J R Soc Med*. 1992; **85**: 605–8.

Lindenfield G. *Managing Anger*. London: Thorsons; 1993.

McClelland DC, Burnham M. Power is the great motivator. *Harvard Business Review*. 1976; **54**(2): 100–10.

Martin V, Rogers AM. *Leading Interprofessional Teams in Health and Social Care*. London: Routledge; 2004.

Maslow AH. A theory of human motivation. *Psychological Review*. 1943; **50**: 370–96.

Mullins LJ. *Management and Organisational Behaviour*. London: Pitman; 2004.

Pareto V. *Translation of Manuale di economia politica (Manual of Political Economy)*. Trans. AS Schwier and AN Page. London: Macmillan; 1971.

Pedler M, Burgoyne J, Boydell T. *A Manager's Guide to Leadership*. Maidenhead: McGraw-Hill Professional; 2004.

Pfeiffer JW, Goodstein LD (eds) *The 1982 Annual of Facilitators, Trainers and Consultants*. San Diego, CA: University Associates; 1982.

Pfeiffer JW, Jones JE (eds). *A Handbook of Structured Experiences for Human Relations Training, Vol. 1 (Revised)*. San Diego, CA: University Associates; 1974.

Rosenberg M. *Nonviolent Communication: a language of life*. Del Mar, CA: PuddleDancer Press; 2003.

Sadler P. *Leadership*. London: Kogan Page; 2003.

Scott RA, Aiken LH, Mechanic D, Moravsic J. Organisational aspects of caring. *Millbank Q*. 1995; **73**: 77–95.

Tooke J. *Aspiring to Excellence*. 2008. Available online at: www.mmcinquiry.org.uk/Final_8_Jan_08_MMC_all.pdf

Wood JC, Wood MC (eds). *J M Juran: critical evaluations in business and management*. Routledge: Abingdon; 2005.

Effective written communication

The aim of this chapter is to provide you with a foundation on which to develop your written communication skills. It covers the role of information in the NHS and the use of information technology in clinical medicine and research. It includes writing memos, medical notes, general reports and a curriculum vitae.

Effective writing

Communication seems easy enough when we talk to people face to face. Yet, mysteriously, those who can charm an audience at a party, when armed with a word processor may use convoluted constructions and obscure words that baffle a reader before the second full stop. Effective writing is the creative use of words in an easily readable form that sends a message from one person to another, accurately and completely. According to Tim Albert, a journalist and trainer who specialised in medical writing and on whose work this information is based, one of the most misleading and pretentious phrases used by scientists is 'in the literature'.

Albert's classic guide *Winning the Publications Game*, now in its third edition (2009), demystifies the process of getting research published in a clear and engaging style. From the initial brief to final manuscript and beyond, all is explained in jargon-free, no-nonsense and encouraging terms. Doctors will find this an essential aid in getting research published. For those of you requiring a quick introduction the following brief notes may help. Should you wish to delve further into this fascinating subject then a study of *Writing on Both Sides of the Brain*, by HA Klauser (1987), is another gem.

The kind of writing dealt with here has nothing to do with pure literature, which is generally written by enthusiasts for themselves, and only rarely considered good enough to be published and shared with others. The writing discussed here is more functional and is concerned mainly with putting messages across, not just out. Medical schools encourage young men and women to reject 'real' English in favour of the particular language of medicine. This is acceptable when communicating with other doctors. When communicating with other people it becomes meaningless gibberish.

Further traps await. Medicine, like all other professions, is highly competitive. Writing is in black and white. Those who have to commit themselves take great care not to offend their peers and, if possible, try to impress upon them the author's grasp of the subject. This is often an effective way of ensuring that the message fails to get through. The all-important principle is to write with your readers' interests in mind at all times. This principle allows for all other rules to be broken. For instance, if the reader will understand better when you split an infinitive (*see* below), you should split one. If the reader has limited knowledge, you should simplify. If the reader needs to come away with a vague or softened message, you should wheel out your euphemisms. Apart from our single principle, there are no absolute, hard-and-fast rules. A written article might need to be revised many times so do not be discouraged if it takes rather longer than you first thought. The word processor has made this easier.

Split infinitives

'Split infinitives' (strictly speaking 'to' plus the infinitive, as an infinitive itself cannot be split) have traditionally been regarded as something to be avoided. Attitudes are now more relaxed, although they should be avoided unless the alternative seems awkward or clumsy. Sometimes splitting the infinitive is clearer than any alternative – 'That was the only way to more than double their involvement.' And sometimes the meaning can be changed – with split – 'Because of the haemorrhage the doctor decided to quickly insert a pack'. Without split – 'Because of the haemorrhage the doctor decided quickly to insert a pack'. Perhaps it is better to rewrite the sentence without the infinitive verb – 'Because of the haemorrhage the doctor inserted a pack at once.'

The process of writing

Planning is useful. Avoid huge undertakings like 'writing a paper' or 'doing a report'. In general, writing can be a laborious business. Break this down into small units, such as 'five possible topics for an article' or the 'headings' for the report. You do not need to be seated at a desk to do this. As Klauser (1987) points out in her excellent book on the process of writing, 'ruminating time' is an essential part of the writing process. The thought you invest at the beginning pays dividends.

The structure and style of a report differs depending on whether it is written for a lay reader or doctor. Writing too much is not a sign that the writer is well informed, but rather that he or she has failed to make basic decisions on what is really important for the audience. And remember your deadline. It should be realistic, allowing ample time for revisions and changes. The best start, as Klauser suggests, is 'mind-mapping'. This involves writing down the elements of the theme on a clean sheet of paper. Then start jotting down questions and thoughts that you will need to deal with, taking them out like the branches of a tree. Buzan (2005, 2006) explains this technique.

Many writers suggest that, wherever possible, you write a first draft of the whole piece in one go. Once you have finished this, put it away for a few days (or at least overnight). When you return to it, relatively fresh, you can start the real work. Leave it for as long as possible, and then start revising.

Active or passive?

If the sentence is written in the passive, the subject receives the action expressed in the verb; that is, the subject is acted upon – 'Findings will be presented by Dr X at the next meeting'. Sentences written in the active are where the subject performs the action expressed in the verb; that is, the subject acts – 'Dr X will present her findings at the next meeting'.

There is a common argument that professional people should not use the first person. However, the passive has three disadvantages: it requires more words, it becomes less vigorous and the writer often fails to state who actually performed the action.

Sometimes the use or overuse of the passive can create awkward sentences, writing that is flat and uninteresting and may even obscure the message. In scientific writing, however, passive voice is more readily accepted since using it allows you to write without using personal pronouns or the names of particular researchers as the subjects of sentences. It also helps to create the appearance of an objective, fact-based discussion because writers can present research and conclusions without attribution. The writing appears to convey information not limited or biased by individual perspectives or personal interests.

The passive does have a place. It is useful when the object of an action is more important than the subject or when causality has yet to be established. And it is also useful when a writer, quite deliberately or for political reasons, wishes to make things unclear.

Writing in the active voice, on the other hand, is one of the most effective ways of improving dense prose. As Gowers (1986), one of the leading authorities on effective style, remarks dryly: 'Overuse of the passive may render a sentence impenetrable.' The active is considered to be a more powerful and straightforward form, using fewer words to convey the same message.

I are indebted to Tim Albert for the following example:

o **Passive:** 'The questionnaires were administered and the results were subsequently analysed. It was discovered after analysis that action was indicated.'

o **Active:** The passive statement above could mean either of the following active alternatives:

   ▸ 'Trained interviewers administered the questionnaires and processed the results. I analysed the figures and concluded that the Director of Public Health had a problem.'

   ▸ 'A work experience student administered the questionnaire and her boyfriend used his computer to process the results. They looked at some of the comments and decided to send them to the *News of the World*.'

General reports

There are frequently 'local' rules that should be followed. These are determined by custom and practice within an organisation or profession. The following are general guidelines that can be adapted to the expectations of the target audience in which your report will be circulated.

- Define the brief carefully and pay attention to the real audience.
- Avoid technical words and jargon.
- Study other reports.
- Pay particular attention to the structure. You will usually have headings and sub-headings. Within each of these sections the usual guidelines apply.
- Use the conclusion to put across the message you wish to stay in the reader's mind. In addition, give a summary, so that busy readers can at least have a quick overview.

Initially, I will deal with the general framework or layout for writing any report. This can apply to a variety of situations in which you may be required to write a report. Examples might include for:

- your employer, possibly after an accident or similar event
- the coroner
- a solicitor
- the police
- a patient's employer or insurance company
- an audit report for your department.

You may be required to write a report either as a lay witness or a professional witness. If you are writing as a lay witness, this means you are writing as a member of the public. If you are the doctor involved in some aspect of the patient's care, you will be asked to provide a report as a professional witness. This is also distinct from writing as an expert witness, both of which are dealt with later in this chapter. There is no right and wrong way: different people have different views and ideas but some general principles emerge. I will deal with general reports first and later with professional and medico-legal reports.

Fact or opinion

I will talk about this more throughout this section, but it needs to be raised here as the majority of reports that you are asked to provide will be statements of fact; that is, giving an account of what took place. And you can and should report only the facts, as you know them. If you are asked to give an opinion, you must only comment within your expertise and in such circumstances should never exceed your level of competence. I will deal with this more fully later in the chapter.

Typical general report

- **Title page:** includes the title and date of the report and the author's name.
- **Contents page:** lists all the main sections and subsections of the report and the pages on which they appear.

o **Acknowledgements:** it is common practice to name and thank sources of help and advice.

o **Aims and objectives/terms of reference:** defines as precisely as possible the purpose for which the report has been prepared and the limits placed on it. Each of these possible section headings has a different meaning: aims are broad statements of intent; objectives are usually stated as 'measurable' outcomes; terms of reference describe precisely the limits placed on the report as well as its aims or objectives.

o **Abstract or summary:** sometimes placed as the front page of the document; this serves to inform the reader of the essence of the whole report in a few words.

o **Summary of conclusions/recommendations:** either or both may be presented at the front of the report. This is dependent on local practice and the nature of the report objectives. They can be presented in tabular or bulleted form and should be as brief and simple as possible.

o **Introduction:** describes briefly the background to the report, the scope and the limitations of the report. The reader should be clear about why the report has been written and, therefore, why it should be worth reading. Tim Albert makes the point that the introduction can be one of two types, a flat introduction –
'This report looks at the future of St Alban's Hospital'
Or one showing the advantage of reading the report –
'This report shows how closing down St Alban's will benefit the local community.'

o **Methods and/or methodology:** often used to describe the same thing, these two words have different meanings. Methods describe the way data was collected. The reasons for selecting one method rather than another should be explained. Methodology requires more fundamental consideration and explanation. Put simply, it is the way the data is used to obtain results and conclusions. It describes an approach to research. Remember you do not take children to the zoology to see the animals.

o **Results or findings:** outcomes and information presented in some sort of logical sequence, dealing perhaps with one area at a time by dividing into three or four further sections. You may include some discussion or opinion in this section but should distinguish between fact and opinion. I have already alluded to the impersonal or personal style of writing. In the past, report writing was very much an impersonal or third-person approach. Indeed many journals will still not consider any other format. There is now a clear move to greater acceptance of the personal approach to writing thoughts and opinions. You must be willing to stand by what you write. The placing of tables, diagrams and graphs is a matter of personal choice. But you are strongly recommended to base this on 'market research'; in other words, look at similar reports – easy when it comes to journal writing but not so easy in an organisational setting – and follow what they do. Apart from anything else the readers will be comfortable with this.

The results or findings can be a good place to include diagrams, tables and the like if they help to clarify the message within the body of the report. If there is too much information, but you believe the reader should be given an opportunity to see it, then put it into an appendix. Always remember the guiding principle – write with the readers' interests in mind at all times.

- **Conclusions:** should emerge from the results and therefore be simply cross-referenced to previous sections so that the reader can easily follow the author's arguments. Conclusions should also only be within the scope of the terms of reference. Avoid introducing something new into the conclusions, which has not been explained previously.
- **Recommendations:** should flow naturally from the report and its conclusions and again cross-referencing enable both author and reader to follow the flow of logic. It is worth considering the 'political' implications of your recommendations, which would require action by others. Perhaps time spent preparing the ground before the report is published would be time well spent.
- **References:** may be placed here as an alternative to within the text. Again, you should be guided by 'research' – and not do just what you feel is right!
- **Bibliography:** sometimes included at this stage, or as an appendix, if the report needs one.
- **Appendices:** start each appendix on a separate page. This section includes graphs, diagrams, charts, statistics, schedules, calculations, plans and source data. Define terms and explain terminology that may be unfamiliar to the target audience.

Summary of important do's and don'ts for reports

Do

- Write your report honestly and don't be influenced by others.
- Write it as soon as possible after the event, while the incident is still fresh in your mind.
- If the report is a result of a complaint or claim, make sure you have seen the complaint or Letter of Claim, or details of any court proceedings, before writing.
- While a medico-legal report should be detailed, as it is better to provide too much information than too little, the opposite might be true for general reports. Many reports fail because they try to put in too much, so don't try to put everything in, but make sure that readers who want to find out more can easily do so: references, websites and appendices are extremely useful devices for overcoming this problem.
- Only include details of events that you personally were involved in.
- Avoid ambiguity and be clear about who did what and when.
- Only include relevant facts; your opinion is only necessary if specifically asked for.
- Write in the first person singular – 'I did this . . .'
- Address the report to the reader you have identified, and avoid jargon and abbreviations that your target reader will not be familiar with.
- Organise the report chronologically – give actual dates, and use either a 24-hour clock to give times, or state whether you are referring to a.m. or p.m.
- Give each incident or event a separate paragraph or section.
- Be objective stating the facts.
- Check spelling, punctuation and grammar before submitting.
- Type, sign and date your report.

○ Keep a copy in your notes and a note of how, when and to whom you submitted it.

Don't

○ Comment on behalf of others, although you can say 'Dr X said . . .'
○ Conceal anything, which will cast doubts on your integrity and make subsequent comments less credible.
○ Make any pejorative, humorous or unnecessary subjective remarks, bearing in mind that a patient or their relatives are likely to see the report.
○ Use the report to criticise others or make general comments on hospital politics.

Supplementary reports and changes

If you are asked to change a report, you should think very carefully about the event before doing this, and only make changes if a factual mistake needs to be rectified. If you have to write a supplementary report to deal with issues that come to light after you have written your original report, make sure that you review your original report, the medical records and any new documentation.

The GMC and writing reports

In their *Good Medical Practice* guide (2006), the GMC give some advice on the probity of writing reports that is applicable also to giving evidence and signing documents. It can be summarised briefly as follows.

○ You must be honest and trustworthy.
○ You must always be honest about your experience, qualifications and position.
○ You must do your best to make sure that any documents you write or sign are not false or misleading.
○ If you have agreed to prepare a report, complete or sign a document or provide evidence, you must do so without unreasonable delay.
○ If you are asked to give evidence or act as a witness in litigation or formal inquiries, you must be honest in all of your spoken and written statements.
○ You must make clear the limits of your knowledge or competence.
○ You must co-operate fully with any formal inquiry into the treatment of a patient and with any complaints procedure that applies to your work.
○ You must disclose to anyone entitled to ask for it any information relevant to an investigation into your own or a colleague's conduct, performance or health. In doing so, you must follow the guidance in *Confidentiality: protecting and providing information* (GMC 2009).
○ You must assist the coroner or procurator fiscal in an inquest or inquiry into a patient's death by responding to their inquiries and by offering all relevant information.
○ You are entitled to remain silent only when your evidence may lead to criminal proceedings being taken against you.

You can read the full advice on the GMC website at www.gmc-uk.org or in *Good Medical Practice* (2006), paragraphs 63–9.

Memos and letters

The most appropriate structure is known as the 'inverted triangle'. Put the important part – the payoff for the reader – in the first sentence. The first few words should not be boring, as in: 'I am in receipt of your letter' or 'The car-parking working party of the senior management group . . . Some people expect a welcoming routine, such as: 'Thank you for your letter' or 'It was good to meet you the other day'. This reinforces our main principle: the interests of the target reader are paramount.

Medical records

It might be useful here to say a few words about medical records, their use, what is included and some important qualities they should have. The GMC says in its guide, *Good Medical Practice* (2006), that

> In providing care you must . . . keep clear, accurate and legible records, reporting the relevant clinical findings, the decisions made, the information given to patients, and any drugs prescribed or other investigation or treatment; make records at the same time as the events you are recording or as soon as possible afterwards.

This should also include referral or follow-up arrangements and, in particular, warnings you may have given patients about requirements for ongoing monitoring, or the consequences of not accepting particular treatments. These events all require good medical records.

Good medical records, electronic or handwritten, are essential for the continuity of care of patients. Adequate medical records enable reliable and accurate recall of each patient's details. They should therefore be comprehensive enough to allow a colleague to carry on where you left off. Indeed, probably the most important reason for maintaining medical records is to ensure continuity of care. They may also be required for legal purposes. For health professionals, good medical records are vital for defending a complaint or clinical negligence claim; they provide a window on the clinical judgement being exercised at the time.

In general, records that are adequate for continuity of care are also sufficiently comprehensive for legal use.

Currently, there is no single model for documenting and communicating information that forms a patient's health record, although healthcare regulatory bodies have provided some standards. In 2005 the NHS Information Standards Board and the three largest regulatory bodies, the General Medical Council, the Nursing and Midwifery Council and the Health professions Council, undertook a review of those existing standards. This resulted in a set of health record and communication practice standards for team-based care that brought together the standards already in existence and common to all three bodies.

The review found that the standards common to all three regulatory bodies fell into four main categories:

○ confidentiality and disclosure

○ communication and information
○ process principles
○ personal and professional knowledge and skills.

They stated that the standards common to all three regulatory bodies were not intended to be best practice but minimum standards to be attained. They are not intended either to replace the standards of the regulatory bodies or any guidance provided by professional organisations. They went on to state that patient safety lies at the heart of clinical governance and the NHS published core standards setting out the level of quality all organisations providing NHS care in England should meet. The standards they identified in the review related to the management of records should be implemented in all NHS organisations. For further information go to www.isb.nhs.uk where there is a section on 'Health Record and Communication Practice Standards for Team Based Care'.

Some basic considerations

The patient to whom the records refer should be identified clearly, with their name and date of birth and NHS or hospital number on each page (or an addressograph label with that information). If your writing is not very legible, type your notes or have them typed. This is a really important point – not enough attention is paid to the fact that written communication fails when it is illegible or ambiguous. Sign and print all entries with your name, date (including the year), time by the 24-hour clock and your status. The entries should be based on the facts you have recorded and written notes as soon as possible after an event.

If information has been given to you by anyone but the patient (e.g. relative, staff member, police, ambulance crew, observer, etc.) record that person's name and position. It should also go without saying that the records should not be altered or amended later; indeed, the records should be such that any attempt to do so should be obvious. Do not leave large gaps between entries or feel tempted to leave space at the bottom of a page to enable you to make a start on a new sheet.

Records should preferably be written in black ink as black colour photocopies well and unlike pencil cannot be altered or rubbed out. It is also claimed that ballpoint pens are less capable of being erased than old-fashioned ink in a fountain pen. The ballpoint also transfers well on carbon copy style forms. Felt-tip pens should be avoided as they tend to bleed through the paper.

According to advice given by medical defence organisations, good medical records should summarise the key details of every patient contact and for the first occasion a patient is seen, records should include:
○ relevant details of the history, including important negatives
○ examination findings, including important negatives
○ differential diagnosis
○ details of any investigations requested and any treatment provided
○ follow-up arrangements
○ what you have told/discussed with the patient.

At follow-up you should also note:

o the patient's progress
o findings on examination
o monitoring and follow-up arrangements
o details of telephone consultations
o details about chaperones present
o any instance in which the patient has refused to be examined or comply with treatment
o record your opinion at the time regarding, for example, diagnosis.

Medical records must be:

o objective recordings of what you have been told or discovered through investigation or examination
o clear and legible
o made contemporaneously, and signed and dated
o kept securely.

Although abbreviations are undoubtedly a great time-saver, you should take care to use them only where their meaning is unambiguous and would be easily understood by your colleagues. Never use abbreviations for making derogatory comments about the patient; for example – SIG (stupid ignorant git), PIN (pain in the neck) and PRATFO (patient reassured and told to 'go away').

The Medical Defence Union (MDU) warned in 2001 in its booklet *Can I See the Records?* that doctors should not make flippant comments about patients in their medical notes, even when they are disguised as acronyms. There was also an article related to this in the *BMJ* (Dobson 2003). While comments may be amusing, they can be misleading, misconstrued, seen as offensive and they certainly will not make a favourable impression if ever read out in court where you may be asked to explain one.

Medical records should contain all the pertinent information about a patient's care and can cover a wide range of material including:

o handwritten notes
o computerised records
o correspondence between health professionals
o laboratory reports
o imaging records, including X-rays
o photographs
o video and other recordings
o printouts from monitoring equipment.

Additions or alterations

If you need to add something to a medical record or make a correction, make sure you enter the date of the amendment and include your name, so no one can accuse you of trying to pass off the amended entry as contemporaneous. Do not obliterate an entry that you wish to correct – run a single line through it so it can still be read.

Patients have the right, under the Data Protection Act (DPA), to ask for factual inaccuracies in the record to be rectified or deleted. The Act does not, however, give them the right to ask for entries expressing professional opinions to be changed. You should only comply with a request if you are satisfied that it is valid (i.e. the entry is indeed factually inaccurate), but if you decide that a correction is not warranted, you should still annotate the disputed entry with the patient's view.

If you decide that the request is valid, add a signed and dated supplementary note to correct the inaccuracy and make it clear that the correction is being made at the patient's request. Avoid deleting the original entry, though. If the patient demands nothing less than deletion, refer them to the Information Commissioner, who will then assess the validity of the request and, if necessary, order the deletion.

Legibility of records

Legibility is a significant problem as research has shown that about 9% of entries are not fully legible, half of all healthcare workers' handwriting is 'poor to fair' and that males over 37 years old were found to have the least legible handwriting. However, there is good news in that bad handwriting is not a characteristic of being a doctor. In fact, tested under the same conditions, doctors are no worse than other health professionals. The difference may lie in the fact that doctors are often under great pressure to write quickly. Furthermore, the consequences of poor legibility are potentially more serious than in many other professions.

Luckily, most GP surgeries have electronic data entry, thus avoiding problems with handwriting, but this is not usually available to hospital doctors. However, computer records are only as good as the person inputting the data, spelling errors can and do occur, and good keyboard skills are necessary to prevent consultations taking longer. And it is unusual for them to be proofread when hard copies are made.

Ownership of medical records

Questions are occasionally raised as to who owns the records and a raft of legislation covers access to medical records. Technically, NHS records belong to the Department of Health and this is taken by some to mean that copyright also belongs to the authorities. In summary, however, the record is owned by the person(s) entering the data, their employing hospital trust or PCT. Fortunately for you, however, in the NHS, applications for access to records are dealt with by the trust. However, your employing trust may be happy for you to deal informally with an approach for access, providing you are comfortable showing a patient their records, the patient is 'competent', it is unlikely to cause serious harm to the patient (e.g. with psychiatric records) and none of the entries in the record relates to another person who has not given their consent.

Access to medical records

Patients have a right of access to their own medical records under the Data Protection Act 1998. If a complaint or claim arises, the records are likely to be examined closely by experts, administrators, lawyers and the courts. Inadequate records that fail to address the key issues will create a poor impression, particularly if they include inappropriate subjective comments about the patient.

Patients can access their records simply by a request to their GP, surgery staff or health authority. It is normal to apply for access in writing. For records held at a hospital, they would normally write to the hospital's patients' services manager or medical records officer. They should receive a response no later than 21 days after an application is received, and by law (Data Protection Act) the hospital or surgery has 40 days to respond to a request in writing. There is usually a charge, £10 for computerised records and up to £50 for manual records, and proof of identity may be requested. The records, when presented to a patient, should be 'in a format they can understand'.

Patients are not allowed access to their records if healthcare professionals believe that information in the records is likely to cause serious harm to the patient or another person or if details about third parties are included in the records, although these may be removed. Patients denied access can approach the Information Commissioner's Office. It is possible to apply to see the records on behalf of someone else with their consent or a power of attorney. For full information go to the government website at www. direct.gov.uk/en/HealthAndWellBeing/HealthServices/ManagingYourHealthcare/ DG_10036450. Also *see* The Patients Association at www.patients-association.org. uk/FAQ-Category/8.

It is also worth knowing that relatives have no automatic rights of access to a patient's medical records, although there may be exceptions with parents/guardians of minors. But be aware that complex family structures may mean that the adult accompanying a child to hospital does not necessarily have parental rights. In Scotland, patients can appoint a proxy decision-maker, who may have access to a patient's records. In all cases of doubt, it is best to speak to a senior colleague or your defence organisation.

It can be very difficult when there are anxious relatives who want to know about a loved one. You must consider your duty of confidentiality to the patient, so you could suggest relatives speak to the patient themselves for information or you could ask the patient how much information they would be happy for relatives to know. Clearly, if the patient cannot be consulted because, perhaps, they are unconscious, you should exercise common sense as it would be insensitive not to consider worried relatives. Occasionally, it might be actively harmful to discuss matters with the patient themselves, and thus it would be in the patient's best interests for you to speak to a relative.

Although there is a duty of confidentiality with regard to medical information on patients, information can be disclosed without consent in the following circumstances:
○ suspected child abuse
○ the patient has a notifiable disease
○ the patient is thought to be an active threat to public safety.

It is advised that you contact your defence association if you are considering disclosing information.

Medical records as legal documents

From a legal point of view most written medical records are considered 'hearsay' and are not deemed admissible in criminal court. They are considered 'business records' if they are contemporaneous, written by the person connected with the events and such records are kept routinely.

Thus medical records may be admissible. However, most legal disputes concern questions of fact where the patient's recollection differs significantly from that of the doctor. Experience suggests that courts have a tendency to believe the memory of a patient, for whom it was a once-in-a-lifetime experience: they will have relived the event countless times and they may also be well geared up for the trial.

The doctor, on the other hand, who may perform many similar procedures daily, may not recall the individual patient and may find it difficult to corroborate events from many years earlier. The doctor's defence relies heavily on the quality of the medical record made at the time.

Therefore, it is important, when discussing operations before patients sign the consent form to not only highlight potential complications but to try to record any conversation verbatim in the notes at the time.

Confidentiality and access

This is a tricky issue and one on which the GMC have issued revised guidance (GMC 2009). Confidentiality tops the list of ethical issues received by the medical defence bodies and the GMC's Standards and Ethics team. This provides guidance on reporting or disclosing information about such issues as:
o   concerns about patients to the Driver and Vehicle Licensing Agency (DVLA)
o   records for financial and administrative purposes
o   gunshot and knife wounds
o   serious communicable diseases (including sexual contacts)
o   issues relating to insurance, employment and similar purposes
o   for education and training purposes
o   responding to criticism in the press.

Visit www.gmc-uk.org/confidentiality for the latest information.

What should medical records contain?

The medical records should include the problem list, the history, the examination, the diagnosis if known, the information given to the patient, details of consent for any interventions required, treatment plans, follow-up arrangements and progress. This allows care to be continued out of normal working hours. It is difficult and wasteful to have to repeat a full clerking every day, but there should be a detailed entry made regularly to update the patient's progress. This is particularly essential before a weekend or bank holiday, when the on-call team are unlikely to know the patient.

It is important that a doctor fills in the medical records as the patient is seen, even perhaps as the consultant is talking. Not all inpatients need daily notes but there should be an entry in the record at least once every 24 hours if they are classified as in 'acute care'. For inpatients in 'rehabilitative care', the minimum recommended standard for review and an entry in the notes is twice per week.

It may not be possible to write in depth when you have 40 patients to see on a post-take ward round. But the following might be regarded as a basic minimum for any entry:

o date and time
o name of senior clinician present
o current problem or diagnosis
o significant changes in clinical status or events since last review
o any significant communication (e.g. patient requests, seen by allied health profes-sional, consent sought or explanations given by medical team, nursing concerns)
o results of any examination made and relevant findings
o significant new test results
o changes in medications or treatment
o planned new investigations
o significant changes to care or management
o a signature and printed name and rank of author, pager 'bleep' number if applicable.

If there has been a recent full summary, and nothing significant has occurred since the last review, and no changes are planned, it can be acceptable to write very little.

The patient's perspective is important and should be recorded in the notes as the patient's personal views. Although the patient's opinion can be written verbatim, limit yours to facts.

I have already stated that patient records should never be altered, but suppose you accidentally write things about patient B in patient A's notes and then realise what you have done! Action should be taken as soon as the error is realised but not by anyone attempting to erase, obliterate or edit notes previously written. Preferably corrections should be by the person who made the original entry. The corrections (and indeed any retrospective entries, and additions) should be clearly marked as such, signed and labelled with the date and time of writing. So draw a single line through the incor-rect entry, write 'written in error', add the date and time, and sign and write your name.

Structure of medical records

Systems often differ from trust to trust and some still follow the principle of having separate notes for each specialty. However, the generally accepted policy currently is that documents within the record should reflect the continuum of patient care, and, therefore, be chronologically set out and not separated into different specialties unless legally required (e.g. HIV information). Records can quickly become confusing and misleading unless a strict order of filing is adhered to and every piece is clearly labelled with at least the patient's name and hospital number.

Most hospitals' record folders have defined places for letters, inpatient entries, outpatient clinic entries and investigations. If this is not followed, information can get lost. This principle of labelling and filing should apply not only to handwritten notes but also to computerised records, correspondence, laboratory reports, images (photographs, videos and X-rays), printouts from monitors (including ECGs) and other charts.

What about discharge summaries?

Published literature suggests that standards are highly variable. In one study 17% of discharge summaries had no diagnosis, 19% no procedure stated and 21% no follow-up. Another published paper suggested that a well-written discharge letter is invaluable to the GP, and 90% of general practitioners feel that a problem list is helpful and that it improves the continuity of care.

Retention of medical records

Finally, what about the time medical records should be retained? In 2009 the Department of Health issued *Records Management: NHS code of practice Parts 1 and 2*, which can be downloaded from www.dh.gov.uk/en/Publicationsandstatistics/ Publications/PublicationsPolicyAndGuidance/DH_4131747.

This is the NHS code of practice and is a guide to the required standards of practice in the management of records for those who work within, or under contract to, NHS organisations in England. It is based on current legal requirements and professional best practice and replaces the old guidance:

o   HSC 1999/053 – For the record
o   HSC 1998/217 – Preservation, retention and destruction of GP records relating to patients
o   HSC 1998/153 – Using electronic patient records in hospitals: Legal requirements and good practice.

The code provides governance arrangements for the NHS. It also states it is an evolving document because standards and practice covered by the code will change over time and will be subject to regular review and updated as necessary.

The guidelines contained in this code of practice apply to NHS records of all types (including records of NHS patients treated on behalf of the NHS in the private healthcare sector) regardless of the media on which they are held.

There are at least 18 large files you can download from the DoH website about medical records if you are so inclined and they would provide hours of reading. But the document *Annex D1: Health Records Retention Schedule* (available at www.dh.gov. uk/en/Publicationsandstatistics/Publications/PublicationsPolicyAndGuidance/ DH_4131747) might be of interest to doctors wondering what to do with any records they have. In previous editions I have summarised the guidelines, giving the minimum retention periods for different categories of patient. In the new Schedule there are 56 pages listing almost 200 types of health record, their minimum retention periods and final action instructions.

This retention schedule details the 'Minimum Retention Period' for each type of health record, although (whatever the media) they may be retained for longer. It says that generally records should not be retained for more than 30 years. Where retention longer than 30 years is thought necessary, perhaps for historical purposes, or pre-1948 records, the National Archives should be consulted.

The following types of record are covered by this retention schedule (regardless of the media on which they are held, including paper, electronic, images and sound, and including all records of NHS patients treated on behalf of the NHS in the private healthcare sector):

o patient health records (electronic or paper-based, including GP medical records)
o records of private patients seen on NHS premises
o Accident & Emergency
o birth and all other registers
o theatre, minor operations and other related registers
o X-ray and imaging reports, output and images
o photographs, slides and other images
o microform (i.e. microfiche/microfilm), audio and video tapes, cassettes, CD-ROMs
o emails
o computerised records
o scanned documents.

The minimum retention periods do vary from as little 48 hours for printouts of operating lists, and a week for request forms: one week, extending through two years for outpatient lists; four years for operating lists in paper format only. At the other end of the scale Creutzfeldt–Jakob disease (CJD) patient records from time of death, forensic medical records, genetic records, homicide and serious 'untoward incident' records, oncology records, request forms that contain clinical information not readily available in health records, standard operating procedures (current and old), blood bank register and blood component audit trail should be retained for 30 years.

Beyond that, personnel health records under occupational surveillance, and personal exposure of an identifiable employee monitoring records should be kept for 40 years; 50 years for records of classified persons under medical surveillance and radiation dose records of classified persons. Permanent retention is required for forensic material in criminal cases and records of destruction of case notes and health records.

At www.connectingforhealth.nhs.uk/systemsandservices/infogov/records you can access a link to a clinicians' guide to record standards by The Royal College of Physicians (RCP) in partnership with NHS Connecting for Health, who developed standards for hospital patient records, approved by the Academy of Medical Royal Colleges. The new standards aim to improve patient safety by standardising the information held on patients throughout their stay in hospital, reducing the likelihood of mistakes and missing information at admission, handover and discharge. You can access this at www.rcplondon.ac.uk/clinical-standards/hiu/medical-records/Pages/Overview.aspx. There you can also download two pdf files on clinicians' guidelines.

o Part 1 has information about current developments in medical record-keeping standards for the Electronic Patient Record. It describes why standards are needed for the structure and content of medical records and how their introduction will affect the work of hospital clinicians.

○ Part 2 contains the new standards plus standard headings and definitions of the hospital Admission Records, and Handover and Discharge Communications.

Summary

Medical records are:

○ a permanent record of the patient's medical history treatment and progress
○ tools facilitating communication between hospital doctors, GPs and other staff
○ a legal document
○ a tool used by hospital quality assurance and audit
○ sometimes to be used for retrospective clinical research.

Medical records should include:

○ handwritten notes
○ correspondence
○ computerised records
○ laboratory reports
○ images (including photographs, videos and X-rays)
○ printouts from monitors (including ECGs)
○ other electrical or electronic charts (e.g. audiograms and tympanograms).

Medical records must be:

○ clear
○ legible
○ identifiable
○ objective
○ contemporaneous
○ first-hand
○ original and unaltered.

Medical Records and the Data Protection Act 1998

Doctors are sometimes puzzled or concerned about case notes, perhaps relating to notes for private patients stored at home or in private rooms. The advice of the Office of Data Protection has stated that anyone who keeps healthcare records, whether they relate to NHS or private patients, must comply with the Act and if any part of the record is held on or has been processed on a computer the doctor is required to register as a 'data controller'. If entirely handwritten, the doctor can choose whether to register or not; the fee is still £35, although an organisation such as a trust with a staff of more than 250 from October 2009 will pay £500.

There is also the question of dealing with the safety of electronically stored data. The relevant section of the Act states: 'appropriate technical and organisational measures shall be taken against unauthorised and unlawful processing of personal data and against accidental loss of, or damage to, personal data'. No manual or electronic system can be 100% secure, but you need to be able to justify what steps you have taken to prevent both theft and unauthorised access.

While paper records are unlikely to be the target of random theft, computer equipment, especially portable equipment, is very vulnerable. As far as unauthorised access is concerned, there will be the question of passwords, although this does not prevent the hard drive from being accessed from another computer, or encryption software. For networked computers there will in addition be the need for firewalls to prevent hackers from gaining access.

Next to consider is the loss of data from hardware or software failure. Various sources suggest that the average life of a computer hard drive is from three to five years, although much depends on how much you use it, how long you leave it on for, whether you carry out regular maintenance and how much care you take to avoid damage such as movement when running. So back-ups will be necessary together with related security. There is also the problem associated with equipment developing faults and requiring maintenance or repairs. Repairs need to be carried out by a reputable company with a written contract that states that the repairer will not attempt to access data.

Finally, there is the question of what to do with old computers. Hard drives are notoriously difficult to erase, even reformatting a hard drive does not make previously held data unrecoverable. There are security products to securely wipe hard drives and companies that specialise in guaranteeing to wipe hard drives.

Copies of the legislation and guides to electronic data are available at a number of sites that can all be accessed via www.the-mdu.com, with 'electronic data' in the search box, but you need to be a member. One useful article on the site discusses reports about breaches of data security by NHS trusts and others, and plans to extend the Data Protection Act, currently being considered by Parliament, have highlighted the importance of professionals being vigilant with their own security arrangements for storage and transfer of patient information and gives advice and guidance. Alternatively, you can access Medical Protection Society (MPS) advice on medical records at www. medicalprotection.org/uk/factsheets/records, and they have a downloadable pdf file from a link at that website.

Medico-legal reports

Medico-legal reporting mostly involves reports on people who have been injured by an accident, either road traffic, industrial or 'slip and trip' accidents in the community. GPs or consultants in a particular field of expertise who assess the injuries provide most reports. These reports try to provide a time-specific prognosis on how long the injuries sustained will take to resolve. GPs in the UK carry out this type of work a lot. Many of the reports involve day-to-day problems as would be experienced in everyday general practice. Some require a specialist opinion and are carried out by consultants, although some reports may be accepted from senior grade doctors with postgraduate qualifications and experience in a particular field of expertise.

At some point in your career, particularly if you work in a specialty dealing with trauma cases, solicitors may request you provide a medical report. You normally have no obligation to write this and may wish to hand it on to a colleague, perhaps someone more senior. As you progress in seniority and acquire more experience you will probably want to write these reports yourself, particularly as they carry a fee. The size of that fee will depend on the complexity of the case and the time and work involved, but the BMA publishes guidelines on such fees and you can always discuss and compare your experience with colleagues locally. Most reputable agencies pay invoices within three to six months after receipt of the report, but solicitors may not pay until the case is settled and that may occasionally take years. So you might want to make your willingness to accept the task conditional on a payment on completion of the report. Indeed a few consultants insist on payment after completion of the report but before submitting it!

Initially, some reading and induction to the provision of reports by an experienced colleague is very much advised. Some doctors approach agencies seeking to carry out this type of work. There are many agencies, from small to very large. Again, seek the advice of your colleagues as to who are the best organised and most reliable agencies.

Most agencies have a template. They are all very similar and along the lines suggested below. This involves a formalised approach to reporting that is logical and enables the insurers and solicitors who view the reports to assess the value of the claim. It does not take long to develop the knack of report writing to a structure. The structure is a great help when seeing the patient to ensure that you have covered everything required.

It can sometimes be helpful to your own thinking in the preparation of a report, and useful to non-medical people reading it, to prepare a chronological order of events that lists exactly what happened and when, including information from typewritten sources (letters, discharge summaries), handwritten medical notes, handwritten nursing records (which often contain information not included elsewhere), and the results of investigations.

The patients are typically seen in a GP practice, private consulting rooms, or even at the individual's home if they have a problem with transport. Remember, if you see them in hospital, the trust may require you to pay a fee for the use of its facilities. Depending on your experience and complexity of the case, the average time to complete the face-to-face consultation is around 30 minutes.

Most solicitors and agencies expect a report to be returned within four to six weeks of instruction being sent to you. You will normally be asked to address a particular issue. This is your 'remit'. Some will require examination of the patient.

Issues in a report you may need to address will include:
- condition
- prognosis
- negligence
- causation.

Your report should be based on:
- the medical records
- your own recollection
- your usual practice

o your history from patient
o your examination of patient
o results of your tests on patient.

Finally, remember your report should be:
o detailed – it is better to provide too much information than too little
o clear – avoid ambiguity and be clear about who did what and when
o objective – only state the facts; it is not an opportunity to criticise others or make comments on hospital politics.

If you have any questions or concerns about what you have been asked to produce, contact your defence society or organisation for further advice.

The medical evidence provided by your report must comply with the requirements of Civil Justice Rules (1998). I recommend, therefore, that before preparing and writing any medico-legal report you obtain a copy of the notes and Part 35 of the Civil Procedure Rules (1998) and the Supplementary Practice Directions.

Try to be proactive with the lawyer who requests the report. Ask questions until you are confident you understand clearly what is being requested. You will need the following:
o hospital records
o X-rays and scans
o general practitioner records
o previous reports
o patient's statement, if appropriate (personal injury cases)
o possibly clinical photographs if not part of hospital records.

Hospitals usually charge for these, so it is normal practice for the solicitor to supply them, or at least copies. Well-organised law firms will supply them in chronological order and paginated. Requests to prepare reports without access to vital materials such as the medical records should always be resisted; it is absolutely essential that the full medical records are sought.

Interpretation of X-rays, etc.
It is said that X-rays and radiological investigations should be reported by radiologists who are familiar with the relevant aspect of radiology, particularly in injury in accidents and paediatric cases. They are more likely to be conversant with normal variants. In practice this means that the films should be seen by an appropriate radiologist. Also it is worth noting that copy films vary in quality, and errors have been made as a result of relying on copy films rather than ensuring that the original films are supplied.

Caution is also required when using routine clinical reports on radiographs. The original request form for the investigation might be very restricted and omit essential clinical information. The report provided by the radiologist at the time may not have been written with forensic investigations or legal proceedings in mind. The author of the report should be approached to clarify matters and given the opportunity to provide further information.

Photographs

It is common for solicitors to fail to provide photographs, sometimes because they do not know of their existence. The nursing section of the hospital records may reveal the fact that a hospital or police photographer visited, and one may have to ask for these photographs to be obtained. Insist on good-quality glossy prints of original photographs, enlarged if necessary, and not make do with laser prints or colour photocopies.

Structuring a medico-legal report

Type the report with double spacing and wide margins. The style and layout can vary, although it is largely determined by the Civil Procedure Rules (1998). It is also influenced by the writer and partly by the needs of the solicitor or barrister. I strongly advise you to be proactive and discuss what is expected from you and look at other reports as examples. You will be required to state the extent of your contact with the patient, the history, symptoms and other details as relevant. Avoid technical jargon unless you give an explanation. Remember that lawyers are interested in the strengths and weaknesses of the case, particularly the latter. Give the results of examinations and investigations and state your opinion with reasons. Distinguish facts from opinions and recognise your assumptions.

Report requirements

The Civil Procedure Rules (1998) specify that the following requirements must be met. The report must:
o be addressed to the court
o set out the substance of your instructions
o include details of any literature or other material relied upon
o state who carried out any test or experiment used for the report and whether or not the test or experiment was carried out under your supervision
o give qualifications of any person who carried out any test or experiment
o summarise any range of opinions and give reasons for your own opinion
o set out a summary of the conclusions
o state that you understand your duty to the court and that you have complied with that duty
o set out the statement of truth in the form required
o give details of your qualifications.

It is helpful to provide a glossary that lists and briefly explains any technical terms used.

Suggested sections

Most of the following suggested sections include statements of fact, but you need to exercise care with those that require opinion. You will most likely not need to include all the suggested sections, which are only listed as guidance.

Summary

A front page with a summary is usually helpful and might include the identity of the patient, the date of the report, date of injury, the cause, the injuries or at least those relevant to your report, treatment and progress, a summary of your examination findings and, finally, the prognosis.

Section 1: Instructions

Describe the source and substance of your instructions and the documents, literature or other material you have seen.

Section 2: Details of claimant

This identifies the patient together with age, sex, date of birth, and age at the time of report of any accident or illness. It is helpful to include subheadings for marital status, family and social history, occupational details and leisure activities. Include a section for other factors which do not fit neatly into other sections but which need a mention.

Section 3: Previous medical history

You should refer particularly to anything relevant to the present symptoms.

Section 4: Present complaints

List the patient's symptoms as precisely as possible.

Section 5: History of injury

Section 6: Treatment

Section 7: Progress of treatment

Section 8: Present examination

Section 9: Investigations

It is important to identify any test or investigation undertaken, the qualifications of the person who carried it out, and whether it was under your supervision.

Section 10: Opinion

This is the most important section and will require careful thought. How do you distinguish facts and opinions? Here are some suggested definitions:

- o **facts** are real and objective
- o **feelings** are emotional responses to situations or events
- o **values** are derived from norms in society, the organisation and the family
- o **opinions** are our personal ideas or explanations about issues, events or situations
- o **assumptions** help to make sense of complexity, but should be distinguished from 'facts'.

In civil proceedings, liability and causation have to be demonstrated on a balance of probabilities. In other words, 'more likely than not'. This could mean a 50.1% chance at least. So the key phrase is 'on the balance of probabilities'. This contrasts with criminal cases, in which the level of proof is generally 'beyond reasonable doubt'.

The Civil Procedure Rules (1998) now require that you summarise any range of opinions as well as giving reasons for your own opinion.

Section 11: Period of incapacity from work or normal activity

Section 12: Period of partial incapacity

Section 13: Residual disability

Section 14: Disfigurement

Section 15: Psychological aspects

Section 16: Special needs

Section 17: Recommendations for treatment and rehabilitation

Section 18: Prognosis and long-term considerations

Section 19: Conclusions
This is distinct from your opinions and should set out a summary of your conclusions, based entirely on the information contained within the report.

Section 20: Compliance with Civil Procedure Rules
Review your report and confirm that you have complied with and understand your duty to the court.

Section 21: Your qualifications
State your qualifications, current post and relevant experience.

Section 22: Data Protection Act 1985
Indicate whether you are retaining the records on a computerised system.

An Appendix or Glossary
Which may be useful in providing explanations of medical jargon and terminology where it has been unavoidable to use them in the report.

Review your report

It is essential that all reports are typed, proofread and signed by you before dispatch. The important features are that the report should be:

○ set out in the form required by the court
○ clearly and concisely written
○ clearly presented
○ clearly structured
○ easy to read.

Each page should be numbered, a header or footer with the patient's name is also useful, and the sections should be numbered for easy reference. Sign and date the report – it is easy to forget this! Your fee note should be separate from the report and not referred to in the report.

Some doctors who prepare few reports do their own word-processing. Others use the services of a medical secretary, who is often familiar with the structure of medical reports. Please read the section on The Data Protection Agency as you might be advised to register (*see* p. 175).

When writing your report, think of the target audience and use plain language, avoiding difficult medical terms.

○ If they have to be used, briefly explain their meaning in lay terms.
○ Keep your sentences short and simple.
○ Check details.
○ Check your facts.
○ If you are writing a long report, break it up into parts with suitable headings.
○ As a medical report is a highly confidential and private document, getting it checked by a third party is not advisable.

Important reminders for medico-legal reports

○ You must comply with the Civil Procedure Rules.
○ Avoid partiality – you are acting as an independent expert. Partiality will compromise your opinion.
○ Never gloss over weaknesses. Better they are revealed early in a case.
○ Do not stray from your area of expertise as you could find yourself challenged later.
○ Make sure you have your patient's consent to disclose their information.

Uncertainty

When writing a report, you may feel or be placed under pressure to express an undue degree of confidence for fear that to do otherwise may weaken a client's case. Regardless of pressure, never be afraid to say that you are simply not sure. 'Unexplained' is an acceptable term that indicates a genuine diagnostic difficulty.

Disclosure of patient information

A report will, more often than not, involve the disclosure of confidential information about a patient. You need to make sure you have the authority to disclose this information, by getting your patient's consent and checking they are clear about the information you will be providing and why it is necessary. Some doctors go as far as to provide the patient with a copy. The MPS Factsheets on Confidentiality give further information about the disclosure of patient information and other defence organisations can provide guidance.

Everyone will read your report

Bear in mind that whatever you write in a medico-legal report can be disclosed. This applies not only to your report but to anything else that you write or say to any of the parties. It is good practice to assume that you will be asked to justify anything that you have said or written. In a report, you should make a point of providing the reasons for having reached particular conclusions.

Limitations in a medico-legal report

There may of necessity be all sorts of limitations to a report in certain situations. Papers or past records may have been unavailable or missing, other reports may be awaited or radiographs supplied may have only been copies rather than originals. Be frank about any limitations.

Report submission

What happens to your report after submission? It usually goes to the patient who checks that the history is correct. It may then be sent to counsel who will consider it and write comments. There may be a meeting or conference of experts at this stage, depending on the size of the case. Later you may be asked to review what you have written, as legal issues are often not identical to medical issues. There is nothing sinister in this, but you should not write something to which you cannot put your name or are not prepared to defend.

The Data Protection Agency

If you are in a practice it is probably already registered with the Government's Data Protection Agency, so this is not an issue. It is again something to discuss with colleagues, but if you are unsure it might be wise to register.

VAT and medical reports

In May 2007 there was another European Court of Justice (ECJ) decision that certain services will no longer be VAT-exempt. Services that will not be VAT-exempt are those that allow a third party to make a decision of a non-therapeutic nature such as:
o reports for solicitors/witness testimony or reports for litigation, compensation or benefit purposes
o signatures on passport applications
o reports or medicals for the purpose of providing certain fitness medical certificates (including heavy goods vehicle [HGV] medicals, pre-employment checks)
o paternity tests
o some occupational health services

o medical negligence claims
o negligence claims whether by examination of the claimant or a review of the notes
o giving an opinion on a person's medical condition for entitlement to pension or disability benefit
o claims by an individual in support of payment of disability pension.

Services that are to protect, maintain or restore the health of an individual will remain VAT-exempt:
o normal medical examinations and procedures
o examinations on behalf of employers or insurance companies
o the taking of blood for tests conducted on behalf of employers or insurance companies
o the provision of certificates of medical fitness, where this service is intended principally to protect the health of the person concerned.
o fees for cremation certificates (forms B, C and F).

If your income from this work exceeds the registration threshold (which is £68,000 pa as of 1 May 2009), you will need to register for VAT and thereafter add VAT to your charges for such services. If your income from this work does not exceed the registration threshold, you need take no action, other than periodically monitoring the situation and registering for VAT if the threshold is exceeded. In reality you are advised to seek the advice of your accountant. You may decide to set up a separate business for your medical report writing.

You can also get the HM Revenue & Customs (HMRC) guide *VAT for Medical Professionals* at www.hmcr.gov.uk/index.htm and an HMRC *List of Services Liable to VAT* at www.hmrc.gov.uk/manuals/vatmanual/vathealth/VATHLT2130.htm (it also gives you a lot more information on VAT relating to adoption and fostering assessments, blood tests, smear tests, character references, reports on fitness to drive, passport signatures, and so on), and an HMRC *VAT Guidance on Changes to Exemption for Medical Services* at www.hmrc.gov.uk/briefs/exempt-med-services.htm.

As well as being obliged to register for VAT, some amendments to your bookkeeping will be necessary. Proper fee note records showing output VAT will have to be maintained, along with proper records of expenditure showing input VAT to be recovered. There are different accounting systems by which VAT is accounted for. Normally, it is quarterly on an invoice raised/received basis. However, an alternative to consider is the 'cash accounting' and 'annual accounting' schemes.

These records will be examined by HMRC regularly, normally shortly after registration and thereafter every three years or so. Any errors in maintaining records or the submission of incorrect VAT returns results in a package of fines and penalties.

For those earning less than £68,000 pa from report writing, registration for VAT is an option. You will need to decide whether the market will bear the additional 17.5 per cent cost of your reports. It may well do so as reports from other experts in other areas already carry VAT. Again your accountant can provide useful advice.

Court appearances

Court appearances are very infrequent and the structure of report writing is designed to eliminate the expense and time involved in a court case. Court is usually a last resort and very uncommon when related to GP reports but may just possibly occur with more specialised cases, although still rarely.

Being an expert witness

A medical expert witness should not be confused with a professional witness. The former provides an expert medical opinion on a case, whereas the latter is requested to testify solely on the observed facts of a case and offer an opinion on those facts. This can be based on written notes and documents, or through an examination of the patient or both. The medical expert is usually not the treating doctor. To become an expert witness doctors put themselves forward as experts and are often chosen from databases of experts held by one of the organisations listed further below.

The medical expert's report or comments must be independent, objective and unbiased. The doctor's expertise helps the court decide the matter before it, although it may be used to diminish the other side's case. It can thus lead to appearing as a witness in court and having the opinion tested by cross-examination. The role can vary from considering a breach of duty in a clinical negligence claim, offering opinions on liability and causation, to examining a claimant and discussing their treatment and what could be offered.

Duties of an expert witness

As in many areas, the GMC provides guidance on the duties of an expert witness whose role is to assist a court on specialist matters within their expertise. The expert's duty to the court overrides any obligation to the person who is instructing or paying them. This means that you have a duty to act independently and not be influenced by the party that retains you. The GMC guidelines on giving expert advice and evidence can be seen in detail at www.gmc-uk.org/guidance/ethical_guidance/expert_witness_guidance.asp#t7, but below is a summary of the most important duties and responsibilities of an expert witness, compiled from many sources.

o Ensure that you understand exactly what questions you are being asked and, if unclear, inadequate or conflicting, seek clarification. If you cannot obtain clear instructions, you should not provide expert advice or opinion.

o When giving evidence or writing reports, restrict your statements to areas in which you have relevant knowledge or experience. You should be aware of the standards and nature of practice at the time of the incident under proceedings.

o Only deal with matters that fall within your professional competence. It is important that you have sufficient experience in the area of expertise. In the event that you are ordered by the court to answer a question, regardless of your expertise, answer to the best of your ability but make clear that you consider the matter to be outside your competence.

○ Act independently of the parties and give a balanced opinion and if there is a range of opinions summarise the range and explain how you arrived at your own view. If you do not have enough information on which to reach a conclusion on a particular point, or your opinion is otherwise qualified, you must make this clear.

○ Express only opinions which you genuinely hold and which are not biased in favour of one particular party.

○ Consider all the material facts in reaching your conclusions.

○ Remember you are not an advocate but solely objective.

○ Do not mislead by omission or omit facts that might detract from a conclusion. Any report you write, or evidence you give, must be accurate, taking reasonable steps to verify any information, and must not deliberately leave out relevant information.

○ State the facts or assumptions on which your opinion is based.

○ Ensure your opinion is properly researched.

○ If insufficient data is available, an opinion should be stated as such.

○ If asked for advice or opinion about an individual without the opportunity to consult or examine them, you should explain any limitations that this may place on your advice or opinion.

○ Avoid misleading opinion that could inhibit proper assessment of a case or lead parties to false views and hopes.

○ Be aware that misleading opinion can also increase costs by requiring competing evidence to be called on issues that should not be contentious.

○ If involved in new research, avoid promoting their findings and avoid subjective bias.

○ Make it clear when a question or issue fails outside your area of expertise.

○ Your advice and evidence will be used by people who do not have a medical background, so you should where possible use language that can be understood by them. You should explain abbreviations and medical and technical terms.

○ If you change your view, you must tell those instructing you, and ensure the opposing party and the judge are aware of this. Usually, you need only inform your instructing solicitor, who will communicate with the other parties. If the solicitor fails to disclose your change of view, you should inform the court. If you are unsure what to do, you should seek legal advice.

○ Be honest, trustworthy, objective and impartial. You must not allow your views about any individual's age, colour, culture, disability, ethnic or national origin, gender, lifestyle, marital or parental status, race, religion or beliefs, sex, sexual orientation or social or economic status to prejudice your evidence or advice.

○ Keep up to date in your specialist area of practice.

○ Ensure you understand, and adhere to, the laws and codes of practice that affect your work as an expert witness.

○ Make sure that you understand how to construct a court-compliant report.

○ Know how to give oral evidence. You are advised to seek training on report writing and courtroom presentation skills.

○ Know the specific framework of law and procedure within which you are working. Proceedings in England, Scotland, Wales and Northern Ireland may be slightly different so you need to familiarise yourself with the process. Sources for this information will be given below.

Guidance on being a witness

Medical Expert Witnesses: guidance from the Academy of Medical Royal Colleges is well worth reading and is available at their website (www.aomrc.org.uk/aomrc/admin/news/docs/AoMRC_Experts1.pdf); it is recent, up to date and concise. In summary it gives guidance to doctors prepared to serve as expert witnesses, but in addition it gives guidance for the legal profession and the courts to assist them in establishing the appropriateness of doctors who serve as expert witnesses. The guidance also points out that the duty of a medical expert witness is to the court rather than to the party who instructs them. Again reference is made to the principles set out in the GMC's *Good Medical Practice*. To fulfil these principles, the medical expert witness should ensure that their statements, reports and verbal evidence are straightforward, rather than intentionally misleading or biased, as objective as possible and not omitting material or information which does not support the opinion expressed or conclusions reached, and properly and fully researched.

The quality and reliability of testimony provided by doctors should be complemented by appropriate professional demeanour. Communication skills of medical expert witnesses should include the careful use of wording that might be regarded as pejorative or pre-judgemental.

Competency to be a witness

The AMRC guidance is also a useful reminder that there is an *Intercollegiate Report on sudden unexpected death in infancy: a multi-agency protocol for care and investigation* (September 2004) that emphasised that it is the responsibility of courts to decide whether a doctor is competent to give evidence as an expert witness and suggests these prompts.

o What is the expert's area of practice?
o Is the doctor still in practice?
o What is the doctor's area of expertise?
o To what extent is the witness an expert in the subject to which the doctor testifies?
o When did the doctor last see a case in their own clinical practice?
o Is the doctor in good standing with their medical royal college?
o Is the doctor up to date with continuing professional development?
o Has the doctor received training in the role of the expert witness in the last five years?
o To what extent is the doctor's view widely held?

Indeed, the AMRC notes recommend that these tests should be applied to all medical expert witnesses. There are some caveats with regard to 'the doctor still in practice'. There could be merit in evidence from a doctor who, though no longer in active practice, can provide testimony relevant to the period during which, say, alleged clinical negligence occurred. In addition, with regard to 'doctor being in good standing with their medical royal college', it notes that not all doctors have medical royal college affiliation. Many non-UK trained doctors are not members or fellows of medical royal colleges and, for these individuals, the 'in good standing' test cannot be applied. Furthermore, 'in good standing' could mean nothing more that being up to date with membership subscriptions and actively participating in a continuing professional development scheme.

Thus, the definition of a doctor as an 'expert' in the context of court proceedings is a matter solely for the court. The mere inclusion of a doctor's name on a list of 'experts' may not be sufficient for the specific aspects of a particular case. Conversely, many doctors not listed in registers or databases of experts may, nevertheless, be sufficiently qualified, trained and experienced to serve as expert witnesses. Several organisations maintain databases or registers of experts with varying degrees of rigour determining eligibility for entry. These include:

o The Academy of Experts at www.academy-experts.org
o The Academy of Medical Royal Colleges at www.aomrc.org.uk
o The Civil Justice Council at www.civiljusticecouncil.gov.uk
o The Expert Witness Institute at www.ewi.org.uk
o The Society of Expert Witnesses at www.sew.org.uk, but you need to be a member to access the website
o The Law Society of Scotland at www.expertwitnessscotland.info/codepract.htm
o British Medical Association (Expert Witness Guidance) at www.bma.org.uk/ap.nsf/Content/Expertwitness, but you need to be a member to access the website
o The UK Register of Expert Witnesses at www.jspubs.com/, but you need to be a member to access the website.

Other useful sources are:
o model forms for reports can be downloaded from www.academy-experts.org/mfer.asp and www.ewi.org.uk
o guidance in being an expert witness at www.aomrc.org.uk and www.ewi.org.uk
o a code of practice for expert witnesses at www.expertwitnessscotland.info/codepract.htm.

The notes also point out that neither the Academy of Medical Royal Colleges nor its constituent Colleges and Faculties operate or endorse registers of expert witnesses, nor do they nominate doctors as experts or vouchsafe those who serve as experts. Finally, the Academy recommends that before agreeing to appear as an expert witness, you should ensure that you understand the responsibilities and duties, best obtained by attending a relevant course or courses approved for CPD. You should also ensure that you have an induction into expert witness work, particularly in those specialties frequently called upon to assist the courts.

Bias

The need to avoid bias has been mentioned several times above and anyone who has ever undertaken any form of serious qualitative research will know that there are at least 17 forms of bias. It therefore requires constant vigilance to avoid bias creeping into a report. For example, reading the medical records of a child with suspected abuse and neglect, you might find that the patient has failed to attend appointments and quite innocently you add this to the list of problems. However, the patient may have kept many others. Someone involved in an RTA might also give a history that leads you to feel they contributed to it. The driver of a car injured in an RTA may have killed a child in the accident. In the first example one has made a point of including negative information without putting it into context. Selective extraction of negative information is one of the most common faults in medical reports. In the latter example personal bias might influence your objectivity. Vigilance and a strong sense of fair play are needed to avoid this trap.

A doctor who is involved in new research should be conscious of the natural tendency to promote their own findings, and should make every attempt to avoid becoming subjectively biased. It is essential that an expert considers and mentions in a report all relevant material, including that which tends to throw some doubt on the expert's conclusion.

Conflicts of interest

The GMC advise that if there is any matter that gives rise to a potential conflict of interest, such as any prior involvement with one of the parties, or a personal interest, you must disclose this, which normally means informing your instructing solicitor. If the solicitor fails to act on this, you should inform the court. If you are at all unsure what to do, you should seek legal advice. You may continue to act as an expert witness only if the court decides that the conflict is not material to the case.

New theories

The place for new medical theories is medical journals and scientific conferences. A court is not the place to float new theories. Doctors who use court cases as a test bed for a new unproven theory do the court a disservice and are inviting complaints from colleagues.

Quoting references from the literature

It may be necessary to refer to the published literature maybe only to show how little data is available. What is not acceptable is to selectively provide a few references that bolster your point of view while ignoring all material that points to a different conclusion. The volume of medical literature is such that one can usually find some articles to support almost any point of view, even an extreme one. The court looks for a balanced assessment of the possibilities.

Disagreement and changing your mind

You may be confronted by the report of a colleague with which you profoundly disagree. Anger or bewilderment is a common reaction. Remember, however, that there is no harm in considering whether it is possible that there is merit in another opinion. However strongly you may feel, do not reject an alternative out of hand; give it consideration, and try to maintain a balanced and professional approach. Legitimate disagreement between colleagues can occur.

If, on reflection, you realise that you have arrived at an incorrect conclusion, it is a strength and not a weakness to acknowledge this. According to David (2004) it is a common experience at experts' meetings that opinions change when one has a chance to better understand the reasoning of a colleague, or when one learns of new facts of which one was unaware. Experts who change their opinions for good reason on receipt of fresh information are respected by the court rather than criticised. However, if you change your opinion, always explain the reasons for the change. Remember, all doctors make mistakes but the most serious error is refusing to admit you have made a mistake, even when it is pointed out.

In child protection cases never, ever consider it in terms of winning or losing. That is something for lawyers, not doctors. The challenge for the doctor writing a report is not to help win a case, but to do a careful, thorough and honest piece of work to the very best of your ability. Remember and take comfort from the fact that the ultimate responsibility for making decisions rests with the court. Interestingly, a High Court judge of the Family Division has also written a useful handbook (Wall 2007) providing simple and practical guidance on all aspects of the duties of experts in child care proceedings.

Things to consider before taking a case as an expert witness

- What is the case about?
- Do you have expertise in this area?
- Could you provide references to support your evidence?
- What are the implications for you if the court does not accept your evidence?
- Are your experience and CV going to support you?
- On whose behalf are you being instructed?
- What is the time scale?
- How much time will be involved?
- Has a fee scale been agreed?

Payment of medical expert witnesses

Research suggests payment varies within the range of £50 per hour up to £200 per hour but, as in many things, fees are under pressure.

Rules and legislation

The rules and laws in respect of appearing as a witness can be obtained from the following sources.

In England and Wales

o The Criminal Justice Act 2003 can be viewed at 'The Criminal Justice Act 2003 can be viewed at www.opsi.gov.uk/acts/acts2003/ukpga_20030044_en_1.
o The Civil Procedure Rules, The Criminal Procedure Rules and The Family Procedure Rules are all available at www.justice.gov.uk/civil/procrules_fin/menus/court_guides.htm.
o Experts in Family Proceedings Relating to Children at www.justice.gov.uk/guidance/docs/Experts.

In Scotland

o The Criminal Procedure Rules and Court Rules can be viewed at www.scotcourts.gov.uk/library/rules/index.asp.

In Northern Ireland

The Rules of the Supreme Court are not available online so you need to contact the Office of Public Sector Information (www.opsi.gov.uk) for details of how to obtain a copy. However, the Criminal Justice (Evidence) (Northern Ireland) Order 2004 is available at www.opsi.gov.uk/SI/si2004/04em1501.htm.

Overriding duty of doctor to the Court

Regardless of whether you are appearing in dealings with civil or criminal proceedings, the overriding duty of the doctor, either in preparing a report or appearing as an expert witness, is to the court and not to any of the parties or the one that instructs.

Professional conduct issues

An article in *Hospital Dr* (Broad 2009) drew attention to some salutary lessons for all medical expert witnesses from the case of Professor Sir Roy Meadow concerning the provision of poor or misleading evidence, or evidence drawn from outside one's expertise. He appeared as an expert witness for the prosecution in several child murder trials and was struck off by the GMC in 2005 after he was found to have offered 'erroneous' and 'misleading' evidence in the Sally Clark case of 1999.

At trial, Meadow said the odds of two children from such an affluent family dying of natural causes were one in 73 million. The Royal Statistical Society later disputed his claim and Clark's conviction was quashed in 2003. Meadow appealed to the High Court, which ruled in his favour in 2006 by a majority decision. The Court of Appeal upheld the High Court decision in part, ruling that Meadow's misconduct was not sufficiently serious to merit the punishment he received.

The Court of Appeal did, however, over turn the High Court's finding that expert witnesses should ordinarily be immune from regulatory bodies' disciplinary hearings. Expert witnesses continue to be immune from civil litigation in respect of the evidence they give.

In 2004, the Deputy Chief Justice was scathing about Munchausen Syndrome by Proxy in setting out the reasons for Angela Cannings' appeal – another mother wrongfully convicted of murdering her child. It led to the overturning of a number of convictions. The law was changed so that no person can be convicted on the basis of expert testimony alone.

Website resources

For more information on being an expert witness visit the following websites.

o BMA Guidance (www.bma.org.uk/employmentandcontracts/2_expert_witnesses). From their website you can download guidance on:
  ‣ information on the licence to practise and revalidation for medical experts
  ‣ report writing and courtroom skills for medical expert witnesses
  ‣ running a medico-legal practice
  ‣ expert witness guidance
  ‣ draft letter from expert witness to instructing solicitors and agencies setting out terms and conditions of appointment
  ‣ preparing professional reports and giving evidence in court
  ‣ response to the Department of Health's consultation *Bearing Good Witness: Proposals for reforming the delivery of medical expert evidence in family law cases*, March 2007.
  But you need to be a member to access them.

o Resources for Victims and Witnesses at the Crown Prosecution Service (CPS) (www.cps.gov.uk/victims_witnesses/resources/).
o Code of Practice and Directory of Expert Witnesses in Scotland ([www.expert witnessscotland.info/](www.expertwitnessscotland.info/)).
o Criminal Procedure and Court Rules in Scotland (www.scotcourts.gov.uk/library/rules/index.asp).
o Bond Solon (www.bondsolon.com) who, as well as being a firm of solicitors, run training programmes.
o The Law Society of England and Wales (www.lawsociety.org.uk/home.law).
o Academy of Medical Royal Colleges (www.aomrc.org.uk).

Getting published

You may also want to read Chapter 7, 'Research'.

Writing journal articles

Getting yourself published is something that adds greatly to your curriculum vitae. You might even make a contribution to your professional colleagues' understanding. Publishing research results in refereed journals is, obviously, most attractive, but it is also difficult. You are unlikely to approach the record of one published medical researcher, Meir Stampfer of Harvard University who, according to *Science Watch Journal*, recently achieved 34,872 citations – surely the world's most prolific medical researcher! You may learn and increase your confidence by getting an article or two accepted by a non-refereed journal. If you are unsure of how to start, ask more senior colleagues to share their experience with you. Having selected a journal, it is essential to obtain a copy of authors' instructions from the publisher. Study the style and approach of examples of previously successful articles before submitting your own.

Creating structure

Here are 10 steps to guide you from initial idea to final article. The actual layout you use will be guided by reference to 'authors' notes' set out by the journal you are aiming at, and also the house style of that journal.

1 Consider all the implications of your idea and ask yourself, 'What am I trying to say?'
2 What do you want a reader to do, say or think after they have read your article? In other words, what are you trying to achieve?
3 Make a plan of the points in your argument to ensure the article flows from point to point.
4 Although normally you might try to capture your reader's interest in the first paragraph, this is not usual for a scientific paper, where the first sentence is very formulaic and dull – and the message is in the last paragraph. (*See* Albert 2009, Chapter 5.)
5 Try to keep your reader's interest by telling them what you are going to say and what you have said.
6 Do not assume others have your level of knowledge, so explain and put them fully in the picture.
7 Discuss, analyse and give reasons for your ideas and arguments.
8 Illustrate by using headings, charts, tables, graphs and pictures, wherever necessary, to clarify and emphasise your points and so break up the text.
9 Summarise and finish by presenting your key conclusions, recommendations and ideas for other readers, prompting further research and discussion.
10 Show a draft to one or more colleagues or friends for comments and honest criticisms then choose the one you want to take notice of because you will inevitably receive contradictory opinions. Ask advice and help from people who have published before.

Common style issues

- When using acronyms, the most common style is to use capitals for each letter pronounced (e.g. BBC and NHSE), otherwise, if pronounced as a single-word acronym, use upper and lower case (e.g. Unesco and Aids).
- Capitals slow the reader down and should be kept to a minimum. Avoid pompous initial capitals as in 'the Doctors', 'the Nurses' but 'the patients'. Words like 'Department', 'Authority' and 'Mission Statement' do not need initial capitals.
- The phrase 'Christian name' is not appropriate in a multiracial society; it is preferable to use 'first name'.
- Exclamation marks should be used extremely sparingly.
- Monologophobia is the fear of using the same word more than once in the same sentence or passage. This fear is overrated and can lead to confusion when, for

example, authors use 'study', 'research', 'analysis' and 'investigation' in one paragraph to describe the same activity.

Some words to avoid/tips

o Amongst – what is wrong with 'among'? Similarly, 'whilst' for 'while'.
o Comprise of – should be 'consist of'.
o Hopefully – not to be used instead of 'I hope' as in: 'Hopefully, the meeting will be good'. Meetings do not have feelings.
o Include – a splendid word for writers because it allows for any complaint that the list is incomplete.
o Try and – should be 'try to'.
o Very – like exclamation marks, use sparingly.
o Quotations – finish with quotation mark before the full stop if not a full sentence.
o Gender – avoid stereotyping; for example, doctors as male and nurses as female. Either use 'his or her' or better still use plural 'their'.
o Methodology – when you mean method. Method is how you do something. Methodology is more than outlining the methods used, although it has been increasingly used as a pretentious substitute for method in scientific and technical contexts. This misuse of methodology obscures an important distinction between the tools of scientific investigation (properly methods) and the principles that determine how such tools are deployed and interpreted.

Overweight words

Try to avoid long words when short ones will do. There are many examples but the following will give you an idea of such words: 'more' instead of 'additional', 'about' for 'approximately', 'very' for 'exceedingly' and 'later' or 'after' instead of 'subsequently'.

Pompous phrases

Again there are numerous examples but the following will demonstrate the principle: 'arrive at a consensus' for 'agree', 'in addition' instead of 'also'. And 'within a short period of time' – what is wrong with 'soon'?

Clichés

These too should be avoided; for example, 'acid test', 'at the end of the day', 'hit the ground running' and 'learning curve'.

Some important points to remember

o Check your spelling and grammar. Nothing spoils credibility more than careless errors. This is the responsibility of the author, not the word processor.
o Avoid padding, which only detracts. Clarity and brevity attract the reader's attention.
o Ensure accuracy.
o Do not make assumptions unless they are clearly stated.
o Check that what you say is justified by evidence from within the report. You may not be there when the reader seeks justification.

○ If a sentence requires a lot of punctuation, break it up into shorter sentences.
○ Limit yourself to one idea per paragraph.
○ Do ask someone else to read it and make comments. The chapters in this book have all been read by at least four people before submission for publication.

Review

Here are 10 questions you could ask yourself about the article after it is written.
1 Is it interesting to read?
2 Is it clearly written?
3 Is it relevant to previous work?
4 Is it built on and relevant to the existing body of knowledge?
5 Is there clear evidence and objectivity?
6 Is there quality and logical progression in your arguments?
7 What are the theoretical and practical implications?
8 Does it meet editorial objectives?
9 Have I left it for a while and then reread it?
10 Have I asked a few others what they think of it?

When your work has been submitted, what will referees look for in your paper? They will consider all the questions set out above. They will also try to identify both strengths and weaknesses of the methods and examine whether the physical measurements, equipment, questionnaires, attitude scales and so on are appropriate to the question posed. Was there a pilot study and data collection to detect any flaws in the design? With the data preparation and analysis, what analysis was required to test the research hypothesis? Is the data at the appropriate level of measurement for the planned statistical tests? Had it received ethics committee approval? Was the methodology appropriate? Could it have been done differently or better?

It is not just the role of those evaluating research to decide whether or not to make changes or innovations based on the findings. As a practising clinician you need to be able to evaluate papers you read in journals that suggest changes in practice. Researchers make an enormous contribution to innovations and changes in practice, but, ultimately, they really only provide the mechanism for that consideration.

Action

Do not expect the skills to come easily, particularly at first. Persevere, and learn from your many mistakes – you will find that you have at your disposal an extremely useful tool. Once you are satisfied with a plan, remind yourself of your brief, arm yourself with your plan and start writing. Most authors on writing suggest that you write the whole piece (or, if it is a long one, a substantial part of it) in one go. This will ensure that the piece is consistent.

Obtain copies of medico-legal reports carried out by more than one experienced person and study the style and layout. Consider the following and decide whether each is fact, feeling, value or opinion.

- Waiting lists are still too high.
- For the third year, despite our best efforts, waiting lists have increased.
- Waiting lists increased by 5% this year compared with last year.
- Waiting lists have increased substantially.

You may also want to consider writing up a case report of an interesting case or unusual presentation you have seen. You will need to do a literature search to ensure that no one has already written up a whole series.

Or you might consider writing up a useful piece of audit you have been involved in, with a message that deserves wider dissemination.

Next time you read a paper in a journal, consider whether there are any flaws in the work. Was it a valid piece of work, logical, well reasoned, etc.?

But the best action you can take is to read the book *Write Effectively* (Albert 2008). It is in effect a writing course set out as a workbook, and is aimed at getting individuals or groups (in learning sets, perhaps) to be able to do the course themselves. You are only reading this book because the author attended a course many years ago, developed an interest and subsequently wrote a number of books.

Writing a curriculum vitae

The last part of this chapter is devoted to a subject that many find daunting and about which I have had many questions in workshops. Perversely, it is now less necessary as deaneries have moved to the new selection procedures discussed in Chapter 3 and Trusts tend to opt for application forms even for consultant posts, although it is a skill worth developing or retaining for occasions when you might need to present a curriculum vitae (CV).

The trend to online applications in many cases now extends to the whole process where you download an application form, complete it and submit it online, sometimes with an attached CV. If you are short-listed and invited for interview the date, place and time for this too will be offered to you online. Therefore, you need to make sure you have a reliable computer and email service.

CVs generally still required

Anecdotal evidence suggests that even with the new selection processes at FT and ST levels, when it comes to an interview many candidates are asked to bring a copy/copies of their current CV, so it remains a useful exercise to keep one up to date. Also some of the better-designed application forms often ask for information in a similar way in which you might have presented it in your CV. So keeping an updated CV on your computer is a useful source of data for filling in these forms as it can act as an *aide-mémoire*.

When the last edition of this book was written CVs were almost universal for the application to a hospital post. But things have changed rapidly and a quick trawl of substantive hospital consultant posts on the *BMJ* online at careers.bmj.com/careers/jobs/view-section.html?action=viewHospitalJobs and also on www.jobs.nhs.uk and for NHS Scotland at www.jobs.scot.nhs.uk/ApplySearch/index.aspx found that out of 100 randomly selected posts 34 required a submission by application form, and 14 of them also required up to 10 copies of your CV. There were 16 still asking only for CVs, of which four requested them by email only. Of the 22 requesting an online application two required a CV in addition. Out of four hospitals that only permitted applications through the NHSJOBS website (www.jobs.nhs.uk), even two of those asked for CVs in addition to the completion of application forms. Interestingly, 20 hospitals asked that you make contact for an informal discussion or visit before applying, so I was unable to determine how the application would proceed from then on. For such visits it would seem advisable to have copies of your CV available.

A similar trawl through general practice partnerships, general medical but non-clinical jobs and international jobs showed that generally though not exclusively CVs are still the normal method of submitting an application.

Applying for jobs

To find the job you want, you need to know and understand the 'market', which varies among specialties. You can do this by attending meetings, talking to people and doing some investigations. Meanwhile, you should be assembling facts for your CV. You need to ask yourself the question: 'Is it the right job for me?' To do so you need the details, job description and person specification. You might also find it useful to talk to others, including your consultants, who know you, the situation generally, the job and the hospital.

Applications for jobs should be clear and concise, typewritten so that they are easy to read, well prepared and presented, accurate and up to date. They may require submission either via an application form or by a CV, or both. An application form has the advantage for the selectors of excluding information not relevant to the application, thereby standardising the process and making it fairer and easier for short-listing. CVs leave more scope for the applicant to show creativity and initiative. The applicant has more control over the selection process by including or excluding information from a CV. Applicants usually prefer CVs. Selectors prefer well-structured standard application forms.

Short-listing panels are generally under time pressure, so help them by being clear and concise and ensuring your CV is typewritten, well prepared, well presented, accurate and up to date. It should include personal details, qualifications, specialty experience, general experience, research and publications. Examination results and honours or distinctions, scholarships, prizes and other awards may be listed. It is usual to give a full list of your degrees and other qualifications with dates awarded under this heading. Always add achievements outside your career.

Keep an eye open for advertisements that state that the closing date will be brought forward if they are overwhelmed by applications. You wouldn't want to miss the job of your dreams.

CV presentation

One way of ensuring that your CV presentation is helpful to the selectors is to set it out in the order of items on the person specification supplied to all candidates. For example, if the person specification was as the example given in the *BMA Guidelines for Good Practice in the Recruitment and Selection of Doctors*, your CV headings would match and be as follows:

○ Personal details
○ Qualifications
○ Clinical Experience
○ Clinical Skills
○ Knowledge
○ Organisation and Planning
○ Teaching
○ Research.

You need to look at the essential and desirable qualities in the person specification in each heading to identify the things to write about, most of which are fairly obvious. Where this is not obvious, for instance in the example quoted, the features of Organisation and Planning include audit, IT skills, experience in teams and understanding of the NHS and resource constraints. You would need to quote such examples of your experience in these areas.

Marital status, number of children and nationality are not required on a CV. Items such as General Medical Council registration number and whether you have right of abode in the UK could be requested and should therefore be included.

Writing your CV is not a process to be hurried. A word processor makes regularly updating your CV very much easier, and unless you do so it is easy to forget publications or other distinctive experience that will enhance your CV.

Follow application instructions

It is important to comply with instructions for applicants sent out by the hospital. Supply the correct number of copies (however unreasonable this may seem). Many hospitals require an application form to be completed. This can be a standard form for all members of staff and may therefore seem inadequate for more senior medical posts due to lack of space. It is always best to complete the form, referring as necessary to the appropriate page of your CV, if you are allowed to submit one, but again be aware that some hospitals state that this practice is not acceptable, in which case you will have to do the best you can with their form. I noticed one hospital that said it would exclude anyone from the short-listing process who submitted a CV.

Application forms can be downloaded from the Internet and it is becoming increasingly common. You can find out more by accessing www.nhs.jobs.nhs.uk. NHS Jobs is the national NHS site for jobs. It is linked with the NHS Careers site for information about careers in the NHS.

Downloaded application forms may be available in a number of ways. As Microsoft Word documents the form can be filled in directly on the computer and any boxes enlarged to take account of the amount written within them. Or they may be written as Adobe pdf files, or as files that can only be printed directly from the computer. Some pdf files can be made to accept text with appropriate software so that you can complete the form on the computer. With the latter forms, software such as Paperport will scan the hard copy of the document and enable you to type directly onto the form. This can transform a handwritten form into a much neater and smarter application form. Check the instructions to ensure that you are not required to complete it by hand.

CV information

There is debate whether previous appointments should be put in chronological or reverse chronological order. Whatever you decide, include a brief summary of your experience. You may also want to classify these under general and specialty experience. Remember that you may need to emphasise certain parts in the light of the requirements of the job for which you are applying.

When listing your publications, accuracy is vitally important. Interviewers occasionally check one or more publications, more for its quality than its existence, and will understandably be unimpressed if they cannot find it. As your publications become more plentiful you may wish to classify them as original papers, abstracts, editorials, chapters in books, books, reviews or letters, etc., and perhaps also note your contribution where there is more than one author. Add posters and presentations at scientific meetings, but only if you delivered the address. Poster displays are often published in abstract form and would thus normally appear under the list of publications, but it is not unreasonable to indicate both under the one heading.

Learned societies and committee membership may include other non-clinical or medical societies if you feel you can justify their inclusion, and committee chairmanship or a period as secretary would indicate managerial experience.

Other interests, whether cultural, sporting or recreational, should be mentioned, especially if they feature distinguishing excellence. Team sports give the impression of team membership and a captaincy may suggest team leadership. Similarly, committee membership of a university or hospital club suggests organisational and administrative ability.

Cover letter and referees

A short covering letter should accompany your application, mentioning the post for which you are applying and stating that you are enclosing copies of your CV if requested and the names of referees. Referees are vital to your application and their choice is therefore important. The choice is still likely to be yours, although there is a trend towards requiring your current educational supervisor or supervising consultant to act as one of your referees. Indeed if you did not include at least one of your current supervising consultants this might be considered unusual. The choice requires considerable thought. They obviously need to think highly enough of you to support your application. Referees now often show you the reference they have written for you and this can be very helpful.

Ask your referees' permission, though, before submitting your application and supply them with copies of the job description and person specification, plus a copy of your CV. Also supply them with the likely date of the interview, so that if they are away at least their secretary will be able to notify the appointing hospital. It reflects badly on a candidate if the named referee has not sent a reference and it may be assumed that the fault lies with the candidate not having allowed sufficient time.

Related reading

Albert T. Effective writing. In: A White (ed.) *Textbook of Management for Doctors*. London: Churchill Livingstone; 1996. (Useful tips on style and grammar.)

Albert T. *A–Z of Medical Writing*. London: BMJ Books; 2000.

Albert T. *Write Effectively: a quick course for busy health workers*. Oxford: Radcliffe Publishing; 2008.

Albert T. *Winning the Publications Game*. 3rd ed. Oxford: Radcliffe Publishing; 2009.

Allison GT. *Essence of Decision: explaining the Cuban Missile Crisis*. Boston, MA: Little, Brown and Company; 1971. (A fascinating insight into meetings at the very highest level and well worth reading in its own right.)

Berwick DM, Winickoff DE. The truth about doctors' handwriting: a prospective study. *BMJ*. 1996; **313**(7072): 1657–8.

BMA. *Guidelines for Good Practice in the Recruitment and Selection of Doctors*. London: British Medical Association; 2000.

BMA. *Career Barriers in Medicine: doctors' experiences*. London: British Medical Association; 2007. Available at: www.bma.org.uk/images/CareerBarriers_tcm41–20743.pdf

BMA. *Junior Doctors Recruitment*. London: British Medical Association; 2008. (You need to be a member to see this document.)

Boyle CM, Young RE, Stevenson JG. Letter: General practitioners' opinions of a new hospital-discharge letter. *Lancet*. 1974; **2**(7878): 466–7.

Broad M. How to become a medical expert witness. HospitalDr.co.uk: guidance. 2009. Available online at: www.hospitaldr.co.uk/guidance/how-to-become-a-medical-expert-witness

Buzan T. *The Ultimate Book of Mind Maps*. London: Thorsons; 2005.

Buzan T. *Use Your Head: innovative learning and thinking techniques to fulfil your potential*. London: BBC Active; 2006.

Buzan T, Buzan B. *The Mind Map Book*. New York: Penguin; 1996.

David TJ. Avoidable pitfalls when writing medical reports for court proceedings in cases of suspected child abuse. *Arch Dis Child*. 2004; **89**: 799–804.

Dobson R. Doctors issue warning over misuse of slang. *BMJ*. 2003; **327**(7411): 360.

Fowler HW. *The New Fowler's Modern English Usage*. 3rd ed. Oxford: Oxford University Press; 2000.

Gatrell J, White T. *Medical Appraisal, Selection and Revalidation*. London: Royal Society of Medicine; 2000.

General Medical Council (GMC). *Confidentiality: protecting and providing information*. London: General Medical Council; 2004.

General Medical Council (GMC). *Good Medical Practice*. London: General Medical Council; 2006.

General Medical Council (GMC). *Confidentiality: supplementary guidance*. London: General Medical Council; 2009.

Goodman NW, Edwards MB, Black A. *Medical Writing: a prescription for clarity*. 3rd ed. Cambridge: Cambridge University Press; 2006.

Gowers E. *The Complete Plain Words*. 3rd ed. Revised by S Greenbaum, J Whitcut. London: HMSO; 1986.

Harris D, Peyton R, Walker M. Teaching in different situations. In: *Training the Trainers: learning and teaching*. London: Royal College of Surgeons; 1996.

Hughes V. *English Language Skills*. London: Macmillan; 1990.

Intercollegiate Report on Sudden Unexpected Death in Infancy: a multi-agency protocol for care and investigation (September 2004) – produced by a working party of the Royal Colleges of Pathologists and of Paediatric and Child Health. The full text is available under 'Publications' at www. rcpath.org

Klauser HA. *Writing on Both Sides of the Brain*. San Francisco, CA: Harper Collins; 1987.

Mann R, Williams J. Standards in medical record keeping. *Clin Med*. 2003; **3**(4): 329–32.

NHSJOBS website at www.nhs.jobs.nhs.uk

NHS Scotland Recruitment website at www.jobs.scot.nhs.uk/ApplySearch/index.aspx

O'Donnell M. *Write for Money: how to do it 2*. London: BMJ Books; 1987.

Paton A. *Write a Paper: how to do it 1*. 2nd ed. London: BMJ Books; 1985.

Report of the Academic Careers Sub-Committee of Modernising Medical Careers and the UK Clinical Research Collaboration. *Medically- and Dentally-Qualified Academic Staff: recommendations for training the researchers and educators of the future*. London: UKCRC and MMC; 2005.

Shortland M, Gregory J. *Communicating Science*. Harlow: Longman; 1991.

Strunk W, White EB. *The Elements of Style*. 4th ed. New York: Macmillan; 1999.

Wall, The Hon. Mr Justice, Hamilton I. *Handbook for Expert Witnesses in Children Act Cases*. 2nd revised ed. Bristol: Jordan Publishing; 2007.

Non-clinical involvement with patients

The aim of this chapter is to guide you through the process of obtaining consent, medical negligence, handling patient complaints and dealing with administrative aspects of post-mortems and coroners' inquests.

Consent

'Consent' is the process by which patients' agreement is obtained by a healthcare professional to provide care. Consent means more than simply getting a signature on a consent form. While there is no English statute setting out the principles of consent, it is a general legal and ethical principle that valid consent must be obtained from the patient before starting any treatment or physical investigation or procedure or providing any personal care. English common law identifies three factors when considering valid consent: competency, information and voluntariness. Case law has established that touching a patient without valid consent could result in action under civil or criminal offence of battery. Should the patient claim lack of knowledge, and he or she suffers harm as a result of treatment, this could be a factor in a claim of negligence against an individual health practitioner.

The patient should, therefore, be given sufficient information to understand the treatment or procedure, and should be fully aware of what can go wrong. Health professionals should also be able to provide evidence that such consent and information has been given. If something is not documented, in a court of law it will generally be assumed that it has not been done. If the basic requirements have not been met and something goes wrong, the door is open for litigation – and the continued growth in litigation is something of which all doctors must be aware.

Case law on consent evolves constantly. Doctors must also be aware that it is their duty, and in their interests, to keep themselves abreast of legal developments. Advice from a senior doctor or lawyer should be sought if you have any doubt about the validity of an intervention. Other legislation affecting consent includes The Human Rights Act 1998, The Human Tissue Act 2004, Human Tissue (Scotland) Act (2006) Mental Capacity Act (2005), Adults with Incapacity (Scotland) 2000, Mental Health Act (2007), Mental Health (Care and Treatment) Scotland Act 2003, Health and Social Care Act 2008, The Family Law Reform Act 1969, The Children's Act 1989 and the Human Fertilisation and Embryology Act 1990.

The principal document for guidance regarding consent for doctors registered with the GMC is *Consent: patients and doctors making decisions together* (GMC 2008). This has replaced the 1998 booklet *Seeking Patients' Consent*. The current version provides a guidance framework which covers the varied situations doctors may face during their careers, including the complex issues with regard to capacity. Serious or persistent failure to follow this guidance could put your registration, and therefore your career, at risk so this small book is an essential addition to your library. This section can only be an introduction to the principles of consent and further information is available on the GMC website.

Seeking consent

You must only seek consent from a patient if you are knowledgeable about the intervention that is proposed. For consent to be valid it has to be given voluntarily by a person (the patient or where relevant another person who has parental responsibility for a patient under 18 years) who has the capacity to give consent.

So, if you are seeking consent you must consider the following.

○ Does the patient have capacity to give consent?
○ Is the consent given voluntarily?
○ Has the patient received sufficient information?
○ Is there a likelihood of additional procedures?
○ What are the associated risks?
○ Are there any alternative treatments?
○ Is there going to be any tissue removed?
○ Is there going to be video recordings or clinical photography?
○ Is the patient going to be involved in any research or innovative treatment?

It is, therefore, quite clear that when you are asked by a senior colleague, or other healthcare professional, to seek informed consent, procedures have to be explained in detail to patients, and you have to be aware of your responsibilities in the event of a positive response to the previous questions. In this situation, theoretical knowledge may not be able to replace practical experience. In the case of more major and complex procedures, consent should therefore be obtained by someone more senior, if only because there can be more complications.

Dealing with patients in obtaining consent provides an important learning opportunity. You must remember that patients may be extremely nervous, very anxious or fearful, and they may not be able to understand the implications of what they are being told.

Many problems can be considered at the time at which you list patients for elective surgery. Many consultants do discuss the procedure with the patient at this stage so it makes sense to obtain consent at the same time, although it is not always clear what patients will need before they come into hospital. There is also the problem of a long wait prior to the admission. It is held as best practice guidance to seek consent again if six months have passed. There is, however, no statute at present to enforce this, in that it is held that valid consent once given has infinite duration. It must be remembered that the patient's condition could change, new information may be available, or the benefit of the proposed intervention may have altered.

Patients can also withhold or withdraw consent – further information is given about these circumstances later in this chapter.

You should use every opportunity possible to develop your skills in dealing with patients at this stage. Ask to sit in with experienced consultants when they have to obtain consent in difficult circumstances. There are certain circumstances where consent cannot be obtained due to the condition of the patient immediately before the procedure is to be carried out, or if an individual is incapable of giving consent.

Emergencies and the temporary incapacity to give consent

An adult who is usually able to give consent can be rendered temporarily incapable to provide consent due to an emergency situation such as a road traffic accident or sudden illness. Unless there are advance refusals of treatment, then a doctor is permitted by law to make interventions which are necessary, and are reasonably required in the patient's best interests. As a general rule, treatment given without consent should be the minimum amount necessary and any treatment which could be reasonably postponed should be delayed until the patient recovers capacity. If there is any doubt about a patient's capacity to make a decision, you must seek legal advice.

Permanent or long-standing incapacity

Where an adult is permanently incapacitated, or if the incapacity is likely to be long-standing, it is lawful to carry out interventions which are in the best interests of the adult. Case law judgements have stated that the patients' best interests extend beyond their medical interests but also covers routine procedures such as basic care, and the provision of nutrition and adequate fluids.

Although it has no validity in court, it is best practice to involve the adult's family or friends closest to him or her in the requirements for the patient to endeavour to achieve a consensus about any treatment, and document it accordingly.

Fluctuating capacity

It is possible that incapacity is transient or can fluctuate. It is therefore good practice to gain consent when the patient is capable, and to remember to also obtain consent in advance for interventions that may be necessary when the adult is incapacitated.

Consent for medical research

The same legal principles apply to obtaining consent for research as to seeking consent for investigations or treatment. The GMC states that particular care should be taken as you must remember that there may be no benefit for the individual to participate in research projects. The patients must be given ample time to think about the implications of the research, and they must never be pressured.

All research projects involving patients will generally have had to receive formal and written approval by the hospital's Ethics Committee.

The same applies to requesting patients' permission to use their medical images in any way. A patient consent form is available on the *BMJ* website.

Children and young people

The legal position for children and young people under the age of 18 years concerning consent (and refusal of treatment) is different to that of adults.

As a general principle consent for the treatment of children of less than 16 years is obtained from an adult holding parental responsibility for the child.

Young people aged 16–17 years are entitled to consent to their own medical treatment. All the same principles pertaining to consent, and to capability to give consent, apply to these young people as they do to adults. However, this consent may be overridden by an adult with parental responsibility, or by a court.

Children under 16 years: the concept of 'Gillick Competence'

Following the case of Gillick v West Norfolk & Wisbech AHA (1986) the concept of 'Gillick Competence' must be understood by all doctors involved in obtaining consent from children.

Following this case the courts have held that children who have the ability to demonstrate sufficient understanding and have the intelligence to understand fully what is involved in a proposed treatment also have the capacity to consent to that treatment, or indeed to refuse treatment.

Junior doctors finding themselves in complex situations should seek advice from their senior colleagues and, if necessary, from legal advisors. Such circumstances are likely to be fraught with distress and emotion, and must be approached with empathy and caution. The legal situation is highly complex, and the courts have significant powers under certain circumstances.

Advance statements/directives (also commonly referred to as a living will)

The purpose of an advance statement/directive is to enable individuals to let people know of their preferences about future medical treatment that they would like to have, or refuse, especially if they are in a condition which prevents them from making their own views known. People who understand the implications of their choice can state in advance how they wish to be treated if they suffer a loss of mental capacity.

All junior and senior doctors have to come to terms with their own response to the statement: 'every adult has the right to consent to or to refuse treatment' – and that includes resuscitation. Many health professionals, particularly doctors and nurses, have considerable difficulty in *not* giving treatment to patients, and struggle with the personal objectives of helping people versus the need to respect each individual's decisions. This is something that you need to consider before you are face to face with these specific situations.

Common law establishes that a decision to receive or refuse treatment made by an adult who has been fully informed and who can understand the implications has the same legal power whether it is spontaneous or made in advance.

The advance statement of a person under 16 years is not legally binding. However, where capacity has been assessed as present, their wishes should be considered.

In order for all decisions to be legally binding, the individual must have envisaged the situation which has subsequently arisen.

There are generally three types of advance statements:

○ one made when an individual is in good health, making a general statement about how they wish to be treated should certain conditions or circumstances arise

○ an advance statement made at a time when an individual is faced with a serious diagnosis, and has various treatment options

○ an advance statement made which nominates a person who should be consulted about an individual's treatment.

If you are consulted by someone who wishes to write an advance statement, you must consider whether there are any reasons to doubt the person's capacity to make the decisions in question. Capacity is assumed unless evidence suggests the contrary. Your signature as a witness may well imply that assessment of capacity has taken place. You must also be aware that a patient cannot demand inappropriate treatment or treatment that is currently illegal, such as euthanasia.

An advance statement may be verbal or written, as long as it is witnessed. It does not have to be witnessed by a doctor.

Will

A will is any properly signed and witnessed document that provides instructions for the disposal of an individual's property after death.

You should never advise a patient as to the content or method of expression within a document intending to be a last will and testament.

If you are asked to act as a witness to a patient's will, you should record this in the patient's health record along with a short note as to the patient's mental capacity at the time. It is advisable that you do not know the patient professionally or personally if you are asked to witness a will.

Do not attempt resuscitation (DNAR) statements and withdrawal of treatment

The information under this heading bears some similarity to that given previously if the DNAR statement is part of an advance statement. However, this often is not the case and the purpose of this section is to provide guidance in the event of having to identify those patients who would not benefit from attempted cardiopulmonary resuscitation (CPR) in the event of arrest.

Good communication is important. The involvement of the patient, those people close to the patient and the entire healthcare team is essential in this process of decision making, as is the communication of those decisions to all the relevant healthcare professionals. Many hospitals have introduced formal DNAR policies and it is wise to be familiar with each hospital's processes.

It is also important to enable your patients to discuss their wishes with you and hospitals are now frequently making written statements available in patient information leaflets, or on wards, to encourage them to do so.

When a DNAR decision has not been recorded in the patient's health record and the precise wishes of the patient/relatives are unknown then CPR should be initiated if cardiac or respiratory arrest occurs. However, this is a general assumption. It is unlikely to be considered unreasonable to attempt to resuscitate a patient who is in the terminal phase of illness or for whom the burden of treatment clearly outweighs the potential benefit.

A DNAR decision should only be made after appropriate consideration of all respects of the patient's condition including likely clinical outcome, the patient's known wishes, patient's human rights (right to life, right to be free from degrading treatment) and the perspectives of all members of the healthcare team.

Patient confidentiality must also be maintained. The views of the patient's relatives and close friends should be considered but these do not have to be determinative. Acknowledgement of the patient's spiritual well-being and religious beliefs is vital, and the healthcare team must facilitate any actions needed to meet the patient's spiritual needs.

The same principles should also apply when a decision is being made about the withdrawal of treatment.

It is preferable that decisions about resuscitation should be made as soon as the diagnosis and prognosis is known rather than at a time of crisis. It is appropriate to consider a DNAR or withdrawal of treatment decision in the following circumstances:
o where the patient's condition indicates that effective CPR is unlikely to be successful
o where CPR is not in accordance with a valid advance directive
o where successful CPR is likely to be followed by a length and quality of life that would not be acceptable to the patient.

A DNAR decision alone applies only to resuscitation so this does not preclude the right of the patient to receive all other treatment and care.

All decisions relating to DNAR and withdrawal of treatment must be recorded in the patient's health record, together with the reasons for the decision and with whom this has been discussed. As with any other aspect of care, decisions must be able to be justified.

All hospitals should have a DNAR alert record system in place and this should be completed. A DNAR decision should be withdrawn if the patient is discharged from hospital, and reconsidered if readmission occurs. DNAR decisions should also be reviewed regularly and the timing of those reviews decided upon conception of the first DNAR statement.

In the case of incapacitated adults, people close to the patient often have the perception that they have the final say about whether CPR is attempted or not. This is not the case, in that doctors have the authority to act in their patient's best interests where valid consent is unavailable. If the clinical decision is seriously challenged, some form of legal view may be necessary.

The use of chaperones

Recent publicity over the practice of some former doctors has raised public concern that chaperones are not being used effectively. This is of most concern in primary care and community settings. Most hospitals have a chaperone policy and this usually states that all patients are entitled to ask for a chaperone to be present for an examination or procedure, although not all requests will be able to be fulfilled. If no chaperone is available, patients have the right to refuse a procedure unless they are not considered able to make a decision and by not having the procedure they would put their life, or someone else's, at risk. Chaperones are most often requested when a male doctor is performing an 'intimate' examination or procedure on a female patient. Research published in the *BMJ* found that male doctors use chaperones in around 68% of cases, and female doctors in only 5% of cases.

The *Guidance on the Role and Effective Use of Chaperones in Primary and Community Care Settings: model chaperone framework*, by the NHS Clinical Governance Support Team (2005) and GMC's *Maintaining Boundaries* (2006) advise that doctors should offer a chaperone for intimate examinations to provide the patient with reassurance and support. Although the presence of one does not provide a doctor with a guarantee of protection against a complaint or legal action, it can certainly discourage unfounded allegations of improper behaviour.

Communication is the key to preparing patients for intimate examinations and the patient must be properly informed of the nature of the examination. The GMC requires that doctors explain to patients why an examination is necessary and what it will involve, giving them the opportunity to ask any questions. The MDU advises that during the examination a doctor may need to further explain what he or she is doing and why. Patients may not understand, for example, why both breasts are examined when a patient complains of a lump in only one.

In *Maintaining Boundaries* (2006), the GMC states that doctors should also record in the patient's notes the discussion about a chaperone and who the chaperone is, or the fact that a chaperone was offered but declined. If either the doctor or the patient wishes a chaperone to be present but none is available, the consultation should be rearranged for a later date where possible. The GMC states that chaperones do not have to be medically qualified and can be a relative or friend of the patient.

But what do you do if a patient refuses a chaperone perhaps wanting few people to know of her complaint even after an explanation that all staff had a duty of confidentiality, and perhaps also refusing to return at a later date with a chaperone of her own choice, saying there was nobody else she wants present and she wants the male doctor to carry out the examination on his own without further delay.

The advice suggests that patients can't be forced to have a chaperone, and doctors must respect patients' right to make their own decisions about medical care. However, the GMC requires doctors to offer one as a matter of course for intimate examinations. The patient's refusal should be recorded in the clinical notes. But the GMC reiterates that the key to preparing patients for intimate examinations is communication, including a full explanation of what is involved in the examination, that patients should have privacy to undress, and the discussion should be kept relevant, avoiding any personal comments.

A model chaperone framework published by the NHS recommends that every primary care organisation should have a chaperone policy and suggests that 'a chaperone is present as a safeguard for all parties (patients and practitioners) and as a witness to the continuing consent of the procedure'.

Advice for intimate examinations

An intimate examination can be stressful and embarrassing for patients, and the GMC regularly receives complaints from patients who feel that doctors have behaved inappropriately during such an examination. The GMC advises that when conducting intimate examinations you should take the following steps.

o Explain to the patient why an examination is necessary and give the patient an opportunity to ask questions.

o Explain what the examination will involve, in a way the patient can understand, so that the patient has a clear idea of what to expect, including any potential pain or discomfort (*see* also previous section on informed consent) or refer to the GMC booklet *Consent: patients and doctors making decisions together* (GMC 2008).

o Obtain the patient's permission before the examination and be prepared to discontinue the examination if the patient asks you to.

o Record in the notes that permission has been obtained.

o Keep the discussion relevant and avoid unnecessary personal comments.

o Offer a chaperone or invite the patient (in advance if possible) to have a relative or friend present.

o If the patient does not want a chaperone, you should record that the offer was made and declined.

o If a chaperone is present, you should record that fact and make a note of the chaperone's identity.

o If for justifiable practical reasons you cannot offer a chaperone, you should explain that to the patient and, if possible, offer to delay the examination to a later date.

o You should record the discussion and its outcome.

o Give the patient privacy to undress and dress and use drapes to maintain the patient's dignity.

o Do not assist the patient in removing clothing unless you have clarified with them that your assistance is required.

The advice also adds that for anaesthetised patients, you must also obtain consent prior to anaesthetisation, usually in writing, for any intimate examination. If you are supervising students you should also ensure that valid consent has been obtained before they carry out any intimate examination under anaesthesia.

Medical negligence

Legal actions in negligence arise when a person who owes a duty of care to another person, because of the relationship which exists between them (for example, a doctor and patient), breaches that duty and causes loss or suffering to occur as a result of the breach. Hospital trusts are vicariously liable for employees' actions carried out in the course of their employment. Doctors are therefore not normally sued directly. Medical defence organisations have no role in litigation against NHS hospitals because from 1990 NHS hospitals began indemnifying their employees against patients' allegations of medical negligence. Trusts thus became defendants in legal proceedings and the NHS accepted financial responsibility for claims. When a patient issues proceedings, the health authority or trust – depending on the date of treatment – is the named defendant.

NHS indemnity provides invaluable support to doctors facing litigation. It is, however, strictly limited in its scope. These limits apply not only to civil litigation. It does not indemnify doctors in respect of disciplinary proceedings within the NHS or brought by the GMC. In the former instance, the relevant NHS body is likely to use its own lawyers to prepare a disciplinary case against a doctor. Criminal proceedings are occasionally undertaken against doctors. The NHS provides no indemnity in such cases, but defence bodies, at their discretion, may be prepared to fund such representation. Doctors providing any private treatment, whether in an NHS hospital or elsewhere, will become a named defendant because they have a legal relationship with the patient separate from NHS indemnity.

So while your NHS indemnity covers you for the consequences of alleged negligence in an NHS hospital or community work in the UK you could be at risk from the following:

o claims arising out of Category 2, work including insurance medical reports, medico-legal reports and signing cremation certificates
o disciplinary procedures by your trust, or the GMC, or an independent hospital
o Good Samaritan acts outside the hospital
o lack of access to 24-hour ethical and medico-legal advice line
o criminal charges as a result of your practice within the NHS.

So it is prudent for doctors to maintain their own indemnity to cover those instances where their employers' indemnity may not help or the employer may even act against them.

Medical defence organisations

The first medical defence organisation was established in 1885 following outrage in the medical community over the case of a Dr David Bradley who was wrongly convicted of a charge of assaulting a woman in his surgery. Although the doctor later received a full pardon, he spent eight months in prison.

Traditionally, medical defence organisations have provided medical indemnity to doctors on either an insured or discretionary basis. An insurance policy is a contractual agreement that will always provide financial assistance under the terms of the policy. Discretionary benefits give a doctor the right to ask for financial support but not necessarily the right to receive it.

Medical defence organisations can help with preventative advice through their advisory, education and risk management services, to reduce the risk of complaints and claims. They can provide the safeguard of defence if you are faced with a claim or complaint. An advisory helpline, in some cases available 24 hours a day, seven days a week, may have in-house legal teams and provide assistance in Good Samaritan acts worldwide.

In 1990 the government introduced National Health Service Indemnity for doctors employed by health authorities or trusts, but defence organisations continue to provide their members with advice and assistance on medico-legal matters including disciplinary charges and complaints.

Medical defence organisations defend the professional reputations of members when their clinical performance is called into question. They may pay legal costs in the civil courts, professional tribunals and criminal courts on behalf of their members. They may also pay compensation to patients who have been harmed by medical negligence during their treatment.

They support members throughout their general professional lives, not just if they face a complaint or claim, as in the following examples.

o Assistance might include advice on confidentiality.
o A solicitor writes requesting to see a patient's notes: should you disclose the information?
o Should you approach the GMC if you are concerned about a colleague's fitness to practise?
o What do you do when a patient refuses to undergo the treatment he/she needs?
o Some have a 24-hour press office to help you deal with inquiries from the media.

The potential size of the problem

The size of clinical negligence compensation within the NHS has grown enormously. To give you some idea of the statistics, in 2008/09, there were 6080 claims of clinical negligence, and the NHS Litigation Authority (NHSLA) received 3743 claims of non-clinical negligence against NHS bodies, up from 5470 claims of clinical negligence and 3380 claims of non-clinical negligence, in 2007/08. £769 million was paid in connection with clinical negligence claims during 2008/09, up from £633 million in 2007/08. As at 31 March 2008, the NHSLA estimated that it had potential liabilities of £4.7 billion. If you want to view the Annual Report and Accounts of the NHSLA go to www.nhsla.com/NR/rdonlyres/3F5DFA84–2463–468B–890C–42C0FC16D4D6/0/NHSLAAnnualReport2008.pdf.

The NHS Litigation Authority

This special health authority was set up in 1995 to oversee the Clinical Negligence Scheme for Trusts (CNST), a voluntary pooling scheme to assist trusts in managing their clinical negligence liabilities. Under NHS indemnity, NHS employers are ordinarily responsible for the negligent acts of their employees where these occur in the course of the NHS employment. The Authority administers four schemes to handle negligence claims against NHS bodies. Three cover clinical claims, while the fourth covers non-clinical incidents, such as accidental injury to visitors or staff. A fifth scheme provides 'first-party' insurance-type cover for NHS bodies' property and expenses.

○ The Clinical Negligence Scheme for Trusts (CNST) is a voluntary membership scheme, to which all NHS trusts, foundation trusts and primary care trusts in England currently belong. It covers all clinical claims where the allegedly negligent incident took place on or after 1 April 1995. The costs of meeting these claims are met through members' contributions on a 'pay-as-you-go' basis.

○ The Existing Liabilities Scheme (ELS) is centrally funded by the Department of Health and covers clinical claims against NHS bodies where the incident took place before April 1995.

○ The Ex-RHAs Scheme is a relatively small scheme covering clinical claims made against the former regional health authorities, which were abolished in 1996. Like the ELS it is centrally funded by the DoH. It differs from the Authority's other schemes in that the Authority is the legal defendant in any action.

○ The Liabilities to Third Parties Scheme (LTPS) and the Property Expenses Scheme (PES), known collectively as the Risk Pooling Schemes for Trusts (RPST), are two voluntary membership schemes covering non-clinical claims where the incident occurred on or after 1 April 1999. Costs are met through members' contributions. The Property Expenses Scheme covers 'first-party' losses by NHS bodies such as property loss or damage.

Currently, fewer than 2% of the cases handled by the NHSLA are litigated in court, with the remainder being settled out of court or abandoned by the claimant. Where appropriate they participate in mediation or other forms of alternative dispute resolution (ADR).

The remit of NHSLA when handling claims against NHS organisations is to 'maximise the resources available for patient care, by defending unjustified actions robustly and settling justified actions efficiently'. They aim to settle claims as promptly as possible and encourage NHS bodies to offer patients explanations and apologies. They try to avoid formal litigation as far as possible and historical data shows that only about 4% of their cases have gone to court, including settlements made on behalf of minors that must be approved by a court.

Clinical Negligence Scheme for Trusts (CNST)

Administered by the NHS Litigation Authority, the CNST provides indemnity to members and their employees in respect of clinical negligence claims arising from events that occurred on or after April 1995. It is funded by contributions paid by member trusts and is often equated to an in-house mutual insurance. The Scheme is for incidents relating to NHS trust employment, and clinicians' own medical defence organisations provide an indemnity in respect of private practice and independent GP and dental practice. In all cases, major or minor, it will be alleged that clinicians have failed to work to a suitably professional standard (the Bolam/Bolitho test) and that, in consequence, the patient has suffered injury and/or loss.

The NHSLA has a panel of specialist solicitors and allocates practices to trusts. Once a panel firm has been instructed, it will represent the interests of the Authority, the member trust, and the trust's employees. One of the objectives set for the NHSLA by Parliament is 'to minimise the overall costs of clinical negligence . . . to the NHS and thus maximise the resources available for patient care by defending unjustified actions robustly and settling justified actions efficiently'. It is for the panel firms, in conjunction with the NHSLA, to assess the chances of a claim succeeding at trial, and the damages likely to be awarded, and then to advise on whether or how the claim should be defended or settled.

The patient is required to prove that the treatment fell below a minimum standard of competence, that he or she has suffered an injury, and it was more likely than not that the injury would have been avoided, or been less severe, with proper treatment.

A claim has to be made within three years of injury, but it can be longer if:

o the patient is a child, when the three-year period only begins on his or her eighteenth birthday
o the patient has a mental disorder within the meaning of the Mental Health Act 1983 so as to be incapable of managing his or her own affairs
o there was an interval before the patient realised or could reasonably have found out that he or she had suffered a significant injury possibly related to his or her treatment
o a court is persuaded that it is fair overall to allow a longer period.

Damages are calculated from two elements. First, from the 'pain, suffering and loss of amenity' caused by the injury. It varies from about £4000 for an unnecessary laparotomy scar, through about £140 000 for blindness to about £200 000 for quadriplegia. The remainder of any award is wholly related to the financial losses and extra expenses caused by the injury.

If you are involved in such a case your role is crucial. The NHSLA need to know what you would say at trial about all the relevant facts so they can work out the chances of the claim succeeding. That might increase the risk of paying too much to settle the claim or going to trial and losing. So they will ask:

o what you did
o the reasoning behind any decision you made
o what your notes say.

They may also ask you to think through what you would have done in a hypothetical situation, remembering that what you think may not be the same for someone outside your field. So you will need to explain even the obvious. However, very few (less than 2%) claims go to trial. Most are settled either by negotiation or mediation.

Lawyers claim they are very conscious of the time taken to resolve claims and this may seem odd to clinicians who routinely have to deal with major problems in minutes or hours. The reasons given for the time taken include the following.

- ○ Time is needed for the condition to stabilise before an accurate valuation on prognosis can be made. This can take years where the claim is on behalf of a young child with a brain injury.
- ○ Time is required for other calls on the time of medical experts. There are frequently issues which cannot be resolved without both parties having had independent expert advice and it is not unusual for respected experts to have an eight to 12-month waiting list.
- ○ It may also take time before a trial date can be allocated.

For further, comprehensive information go to www.nhsla.com/home.htm where you will also find a link to 'advice for clinicians'.

Action for Victims of Medical Accidents (AVMA)

AVMA, founded in 1982, provides independent advice and support to patients injured and harmed during the course of medical treatment. It has been suggested that an estimated 850 000 medical errors occur in NHS hospitals every year resulting in 40 000 deaths (Aylin *et al.* 2004). AVMA is a charitable organisation and employs a team of medically trained caseworkers and support staff to help patients with their complaints about medical treatment. AVMA also works closely with selected members of the legal profession and occupies a unique position in the field of medical accidents since it is authorised by the Legal Services Commission (formally the Legal Aid Board) to accredit and monitor selected solicitors in the field of clinical negligence. For more information visit the AVMA website at www.avma.org.uk.

Children and bereavement

Children who are forewarned of the imminence and inevitability of someone's death have lower anxiety levels as a result than those who are not forewarned. Young children are often said to need the concrete experience of seeing the parent after death. The bereaved adult may find this difficult and the doctor may be able to offer to accompany the child. Further counselling is normally the responsibility of the primary care team using appropriate counselling services as required. Cruse – the national charity for bereavement care – publishes literature for bereaved children and their carers as well as providing training and counselling services. The Macmillan Children's Bereavement Service provides help for children and young people to talk about bereavement or a life limiting illness.

According to the BBC News and Information website (May 2004), a child is bereaved of a parent every 30 minutes in Britain, one in three loses a sibling during childhood and 70% of schools are expected to deal with related problems. The

National Children's Bureau says teachers are often afraid of saying the wrong thing and has called for issues surrounding death to become part of science and religious studies lessons. The NCB has written a booklet (*Childhood Bereavement: developing the curriculum and pastoral support* [Job 2004]) of advice for schools that recommends ignoring euphemisms, such as 'passed away' and 'sleeping', for fear children will think the deceased parent is going to return. Sometimes children and young people want to talk openly about their loss, but find that it is those around them that avoid the issue.

For those requiring more on this subject I would refer you to the related reading list at the end of this chapter.

Last offices

A last office is the care given to a person who has died. It should demonstrate respect for the dead, should be carried out with privacy and dignity, and must be focused on fulfilling cultural and religious beliefs and traditions. It also has to comply with legal and health and safety requirements.

It is unusual for doctors to be directly involved in the performing of last offices, as it has traditionally been a nursing role. Many nurses view this task with symbolic significance as it is the final demonstration of care given to the patient, and this should be respected by doctors. Last offices also give the family the message that care continues even after death. It is, however, crucial that doctors are aware of legal requirements for the care of the dead, and the correct procedures to be followed.

Some hospitals have taken the last offices procedure away from hospitals, giving the responsibility to the undertakers or the mortuary. This can cause difficulties for staff in following some cultural and religious processes. There are end of life care tools such as the Liverpool Care Pathway for the Dying (Ellershaw and Wilkinson 2003) which asserts practices – legal, removal of defunct invasive equipment, ensuring correct identification for example – for the care of the dying and care after death.

Death and religion

Behaviour which is in ignorance of the religious beliefs and needs of a dying patient and relatives may cause great distress and offence. The following are only guidelines as there are wide variations within all the world's faiths. Problems are likely to occur with patients whose cultures and beliefs differ considerably from those of your own religion. If in doubt, consult the family or use the contacts listed below. In many cultures, grief is expressed more openly than in the West and wherever possible a side ward should be made available to allow families and friends time with the deceased if they wish. Jewellery and insignia of possible religious significance should not be removed from the body without the permission of the relatives. It is, of course, imperative that the bodies of those belonging to any religious sect are treated with respect and dignity according to any traditions.

Baha'i

o The body of the deceased should be treated with respect. Baha'i relatives may wish to say prayers for the deceased person.
o Normal last offices may be performed by the nursing staff.
o Baha'i adherents may not be cremated, nor may they be buried more than an hour's journey from the place of death.
o A special ring will be placed on the finger of the deceased and must not be removed.
o Baha'is have no objection to post-mortem examination and may leave their bodies to scientific research or may donate organs if they so wish.
o Further information can be obtained from the National Spiritual Assembly of the Baha'is of the UK, Tel: 020 7590 8792, or go to www.bahai.org.uk.

Buddhism

o There is no prescribed ritual for the handling of the body of a Buddhist person so customary last offices are appropriate.
o A request for a Buddhist monk or nun to be present may be made.
o There is a number of schools of Buddhism – relatives should be contacted for advice as sects may have strong views on how the body should be treated.
o When the person dies, the monk or nun should be informed (the relatives often do this) and the body should not be moved for one hour after death.
o There are unlikely to be objections to post-mortem examination or organ donation – although some Far Eastern Buddhists may object to this.
o The patient's body should be wrapped in an unmarked sheet.
o For further information contact The Buddhist Hospice Trust, 1 Laurel House, Trafalgar Square, Newport, Isle of Wight. Tel: 01983 526945.

Christianity

o There are many denominations and degrees of adherence with the Christian faith. In most cases customary last offices are acceptable.
o Relatives may wish staff to call the hospital chaplain, or minister or priest from their own church to either perform last rites, say prayers or give Holy Communion. The last may be held with family members also taking communion.
o Some Roman Catholics may wish to place a rosary in the patient's hands, and/or a crucifix at the patient's head.
o Some Christian Orthodox families may wish to place an icon at either side of the patient's head.
o For further information consult the hospital chaplain or local denominational minister.
o The Free Church and Church of Scotland have different practices so check with relatives.
o A useful website is www.nhs-chaplaincy-spiritualcare.org.uk.
o Quakers (The Religious Society of Friends) have no clergy but the presence of another Quaker or the hospital chaplain is usually acceptable.

Hinduism

○ If required by relatives, inform the family priest or one from the local temple. Relatives may wish to read from the Bhagavad-Gita or make a request that staff read extracts during last offices.

○ The family may wish to assist in last offices and may request that the patient is dressed in their own clothes. If possible the eldest son should be present. Relatives of the same sex as the patient may wish to wash the body, preferably in water mixed with water from the River Ganges.

○ A Hindu may like to have leaves of the sacred tulsi plant and Ganges water placed in his or her mouth by relatives before death. It is therefore very important to inform relatives that death is imminent.

○ If no relatives are there, staff of the same sex as the patient should wear gloves and apron, straighten the body, close the eyes and support the jaw before wrapping in a sheet. The body should not be washed. Jewellery or sacred threads must not be removed.

○ The patient's family may request that the patient be placed on the floor and they may wish to burn incense.

○ The patient is usually cremated as soon as possible after death.

○ Post-mortems are viewed as disrespectful to the deceased person, so are only carried out when strictly necessary.

○ For further information contact the nearest Hindu temple (*see* telephone directory), or go to www.hinducouncil.uk.org.

Humanism

○ Humanism is not a religion but a rationalist non-religious approach to life.

○ Individuals who define themselves as Humanists should be involved as much as possible, like all patients, in what happens to them before and after death.

Jainism

○ Relatives may wish to contact their priest to recite prayers with the patient and family.

○ The family may wish to be present or to help with the last offices.

○ The family may ask for the patient to be clothed in a plain white gown (which they may supply), and then wrapped in a plain white sheet.

○ Post-mortems may be seen as disrespectful, depending on the degree of orthodoxy of the patient.

○ Organ donation is acceptable.

○ Cremation is arranged whenever possible within 24 hours of death.

○ Orthodox Jains may have chosen the path of Selleklana, which is death by ritual fasting. This is rarely practised today but may still have an influence on the Jain attitude to death.

○ For further information contact The Institute of Jainology, Tel: 020 8997 2300 or the Jain Centre, Tel: 0116 254 3091, or go to www.jainism.org.

Jehovah's Witnesses

- Routine last offices are appropriate. Relatives may wish to be present, and may read from the bible or pray.
- The family will inform staff should there be any special requirements, which may vary depending on the patient's country of origin.
- Post-mortem examinations will be refused unless absolutely necessary.
- Organ donations may be acceptable.
- Further information may be obtained from the nearest Kingdom Hall (telephone directory) or the Watch Tower Bible & Tract Society (Medical Desk), Tel: 020 8906 2211.

Judaism

- The family will contact their own rabbi, or the hospital chaplain will advise.
- Prayers may be recited by those present.
- Traditionally the body is left for eight minutes before being moved. A feather may be placed over the lips and nose to detect signs of breath.
- Staff members are permitted to perform procedures for preserving dignity and honour. The body must be handled as little as possible, and staff must wear gloves. The body must not be washed. Staff may straighten the body, leaving the arms parallel and close to the body with the hands open.
- Bodies must remain in the clothes in which they died. The body will be washed by the Holy Assembly, which performs a ritual purification.
- Watchers stay with the body until burial (normally within 24 hours). In this period a quiet non-denominational room is appreciated, where the body can be placed with its feet towards the door.
- If death occurs on the Sabbath (sunset Friday to sunset Saturday), watchers will remain with the body until the Sabbath is over, as funerals cannot take place during this time.
- In some areas, the Registrars Office will arrange to be open on Sundays and Bank Holidays to allow for registration of death.
- Post-mortems are only permitted if required by law.
- Organ donation is sometimes permitted.
- Burial is preferred but non-orthodox Jews may choose to be cremated.
- Further information may be obtained from The Burial Society of the United Synagogue, Tel: 020 8343 3456 or the Office of the Chief Rabbi (Orthodox), Tel: 020 8343 6301.

Mormon (Church of Jesus Christ of the Latter Day Saints)

- No special requirements.
- Relatives may wish to be at last offices.
- Relatives will advise if the patient wears one or two-piece sacred undergarment; if so, they will dress the patient as necessary.
- For further information contact the local church or the Head Office, Tel: 0121 712 1200, or go to www.ldschurch.org.

Muslim (Islam)

o Where possible the bed should be turned so that the body is facing Mecca. If the bed cannot be moved the patient should be turned onto their right sides so their face is towards Mecca.
o Muslims may object to the body being touched by someone of a different faith or opposite sex. If no family is present, staff must wear gloves to close eyes, straighten body, support jaw and turn the head to the right shoulder.
o The body must not be washed or nails cut.
o The body should be covered in a plain white sheet.
o Cremation is forbidden.
o Burial takes place within 24 hours wherever possible.
o The body is normally taken home or to a mosque where it is washed by another Muslim of the same sex.
o Post-mortems are only permitted if required by law.
o Organ donation is not always encouraged, although a Fatwa (religious verdict) has been issued by UK Muslim Law Council which allows Muslims to donate.
o Further information from IQRA Trust, Tel: 020 7838 7987, or go to www.iqratrust. org.uk.

Rastafarian

o Usual last offices are permitted, although the patient's family may like to be present to say prayers.
o Post-mortems are refused unless absolutely necessary.
o Permission for organ donation is unlikely.
o For further information, or go to www.rastafarian.net.

Sikhism

o Family members, especially the eldest son, and friends will be present if able.
o Usually families will perform last offices, but staff may straighten the body, close the eyes and support the jaw and wrap it in a clean white sheet.
o The '5ks' must not be removed; these are personal items sacred to a Sikh:
  ‣ Kesh: do not cut hair or beard or remove turban
  ‣ Kanga: do not remove semi-circular comb which fixes the uncut hair
  ‣ Kara: do not remove bracelet from the wrist
  ‣ Kaccha: do not remove the special shorts worn as underwear
  ‣ Kirpan: do not remove the sword (usually miniature).
o The family will wash and dress the patient's body.
o Post-mortems will be refused unless required by law.
o Sikhs are always cremated.
o Organ donation is permitted but is rare as they do not wish the body to be mutilated.
o For further information contact the nearest Sikh temple or the Sikh Missionary Society UK, Tel: 020 8574 1902, or go to www.bbc.co.uk/religion/religions/ sikhism.

Zoroastrian (Parsee)

○ Usually, normal last offices are permitted. The family may wish to be present or to participate.
○ Orthodox Parsees require a priest to be present if possible.
○ After washing, the body is dressed in the Sadra (white cotton or muslin) and Kusti, which is a girdle woven of 72 strands of lamb's wool symbolising the 72 chapters of the Yasna (liturgy).
○ The head may be covered with a white cap or scarf.
○ The funeral will take place as soon as possible after death.
○ Burial or cremation is acceptable.
○ Post-mortems are forbidden unless required by law.
○ Organ donation is forbidden.
○ Further information may be obtained from the Zoroastrian Trust Funds of Europe. Tel: 020 8866 0765, or go to www.bbc.co.u./religion/religions/zoroastrian.

Helping or counselling

Nursing staff are helpful in advising bereaved relatives on the procedures for registration of death, cremation certificates and finding a suitable undertaker. The hospital chaplain may take on these duties and may be able to put relatives in touch with members of their own religion or community when no relatives are easily accessible.

Death, certification and cremation

There are currently three categories of death:
○ those certified by a doctor
○ those certified by a doctor with the coroner's agreement
○ those reported to and investigated by the coroner.

When a death is reported to the coroner they may: certify the death on the basis of the information they have available or have acquired; or certify the death after ordering an autopsy; or even certify the death after holding an inquest (of which more below).

However, in the draft legislative programme of the government for 2009 is a proposed Coroners and Death Certification Bill. The purpose of this Bill is provide a new system of death investigation for families, so that they can be assured that the cause of death of their relative has been properly established and that, where possible, lessons can be learned to prevent future deaths. The main elements of the Bill are to:
○ create a new national coroner service, moving towards fulltime coroners working to national minimum standards (funding responsibility will remain with local authorities)
○ create a new system of secondary certification of deaths that are not referred to the coroner, covering both burials and cremations
○ establish a new group of medical examiners to scrutinise independently the causes of death given by doctors on death certificates

o introduce new powers of investigation for coroners, including improved procedures for post-mortems and inquests

o establish a new Chief Coroner as head of the coroner service, improve arrangements for coroner appointments and training, and provide for independent inspection of coroners

o create new flexible boundaries between coroner areas to enable services to be delivered to families more effectively, and with powers for the Chief Coroner to reallocate work to prevent backlogs of work developing

o establish new and accessible rights of appeal for bereaved people against coroners' decisions

o introduce a Charter for the Bereaved outlining a full range of rights for bereaved people to be informed and consulted about case progress by coroners.

So this section may not remain an accurate overview of the current system. It should also be noted that there are variations in interpretation between individual coroners and crematoria, and indeed trusts are likely to have policies for dealing with the death of a patient. The practice outside England and Wales may show differences, although much also applies to Scotland and the Procurator Fiscal. If you are a member of the MDU you can read about the rules in Scotland and Wales by going to www.the-mdu.com.

It might be helpful to highlight one or two common misconceptions. Death certification is not the same as verification of death. Depending on circumstances, a number of individuals other than doctors can confirm a death including a senior nurse or paramedic. A doctor who has attended the deceased during the last illness and who has seen the deceased in the last 14 days is normally required to issue the Medical Certificate of Cause of Death (MCCD). This is often known as certifying death and in hospital could be done by any member of the medical team, and outside hospital usually the GP of the deceased. A doctor not in attendance during the last 14 days of illness may also certify provided they attended the last illness and have seen the body after death or have the coroner's permission.

Requesting a post-mortem

There are two possible reasons for requesting a post-mortem. The first arises as a statutory requirement if a coroner's inquest is to be held. The second is when it is felt that significant benefit would be gained from further investigation into the cause of death. Several studies have shown that even when patients have been intensively investigated in hospital, the cause of death is wrong in about 10–15% of cases, with major unexpected conditions in up to 75% of cases. Furthermore doctors have been shown to be poor at predicting those cases likely to exhibit unexpected findings.

Some communication skills, such as the breaking of bad news, are transferable between different areas of clinical practice. Autopsy requests represent a specific requirement for communication skills training that is probably not transferable and therefore requires specific attention.

Even clinicians with little or no interest in autopsies may still have to inform relatives of the requirement for a medico-legal autopsy and all clinicians should therefore be capable of providing adequate reassurance regarding the autopsy to bereaved relatives. It is often clinicians who cannot provide adequate reassurance regarding the fears and reservations expressed by relatives that makes them reluctant to request autopsies because of the personal discomfort experienced when approaching bereaved relatives for consent.

The process of requesting an autopsy from recently bereaved relatives is stressful for doctors and any sense of personal discomfort will decrease the motivation of clinicians to request autopsies. This difficult request of relatives often falls to junior staff. A request for a post-mortem is of necessity made at a time of grief and distress for relatives, especially as they tend to be associated with a bereavement which is sudden, unexpected or traumatic. There is likely therefore to be denial, perhaps dissociation, in addition to the grief. The relatives' mental state may understandably be difficult to deal with thus you may encounter anger, resentment or rejection.

Many studies have highlighted the problems of obtaining permission for autopsies and most clinicians have no formal training in how to obtain permission. Studies have also shown that provision of training in how to request permission for autopsies has contributed to the improvement of autopsy rates. Those clinicians who have received appropriate training have more confidence and consequently may be more willing to take the time to educate relatives in the nature and the importance of the autopsy. The manner in which permission for autopsy is sought is important and can in some cases influence the decision of the family.

Although formal training is thought to be appropriate between the beginning of the final undergraduate year and the end of the pre-registration house officer year, some further assistance is useful later. Active methods, such as demonstration video sessions, video feedback sessions based on the performance of participants and role-play techniques, have been found to be more desirable than the more passive training methods such as written guidelines and lectures. Your local trust may well provide such opportunities.

It may be better to break the bad news separately from the gaining of permission for a post-mortem. You also need to agree who is going to do it and who you are going to ask for permission.

Key people involved with agreeing post-mortems

The doctor

Breaking bad news is difficult enough for any doctor, but having to deal with distressed relatives and give bad news is a significant stress for all doctors. Being less experienced and less senior adds to that stress. The difficulty of requesting a post-mortem adds further to the stress.

It is easy to think that your main task is to get permission. But that takes no account of your personal attitude to dying, death and post-mortem examination to say nothing of your feelings about what a post-mortem may say of the correct diagnosis, which may reveal errors in earlier diagnosis and treatment.

Although the responsibility for obtaining consent is often passed to more junior doctors, ultimately it is the responsibility of the consultant. It is important, however, that the doctor making the request should have sufficient knowledge of the case and procedure to inform the relatives and answer any of their questions adequately. Trusts often have policies on this issue and may specify the grade of doctor making such a request. Some trusts have bereavement officers responsible for these policies.

Family members

It is also easy to forget in the emotionally charged atmosphere that the family may want answers too, not for any reason of possible litigation but in the natural desire to know why, what happened, and how it happened.

Relatives and family will have personal, religious and cultural attitudes towards death and medical science. They may have a fear about the body being cut up, that their relative may not really be dead. A poorly handled request for a post-mortem can be a source of additional stress to relatives. In some cases, although a full post-mortem may be ideal, the next of kin may impose limitations, such as the head not being opened, or examination limited to certain organs, maybe heart or lungs or specific areas such as the abdomen or chest. The next of kin can also specify whether material may be kept for histology, teaching or research.

The pathologist

This is not a two-party process but a triangle with the person carrying out the post-mortem involved too. It can be easy for them to forget about their colleagues who have to discuss issues face to face with relatives. Delays in getting results to medical staff can be frustrating, contribute to tensions and be worrying. For relatives, the delays can be agonising.

The approach

The individual approach of the doctor can be helpful and soften the blow, whereas for others this may exacerbate the emotional trauma for relatives. Relatives seem to gain support when they perceive that the informant is also distressed. A cold, impersonal, 'professional' approach might even cause offence. There are basically three ways of approaching the problem:

o blunt and insensitive – accepting that relatives will be upset whatever is said
o kind and sad – but without any positive support or encouragement or optimism
o understanding and positive – with flexibility, reassurance and empathy.

The right approach is obvious, but you will be aware that there are many complicating factors – most of which I hope we have covered in the preceding sections.

Making the request

In olden times, messengers bringing news of battles lost were often executed. There is still a tendency to blame a messenger for bad news. Doctors are no exception. Patients and doctors often harbour unrealistic expectations about modern medicine. Guidelines for breaking bad news are relevant here (*see* p. 83).

People respond according to their personality, which is often difficult to predict. Stunned silence, disbelief, guilt, anger, acute stress can all occur. Anger and acute stress are especially problematic, but stunned silence and disbelief are also difficult. Anger may be directed at the doctor, the medical profession, medical science, the hospital or at the NHS in general, but meeting this with anger only exacerbates the situation.

Allowing the relative to cry can be important to them. People value doctors who can cope with tears without being embarrassed. The doctor's instinctive reaction is usually to treat tears like haemorrhage – stop them as quickly as possible. Doctors should be able to display emotion, particularly as cool professional detachment can so easily be interpreted as evasive and unsympathetic.

Remember that the most difficult aspects for the clinician are often not those of most concern to the relative, so it is important to check continually on the responses and feelings of a relative and allow time and opportunities for things to sink in and think about questions.

Reporting cases to the coroner

As already indicated, at the time of writing the whole system of 'Death, Certification, Coroner and Cremation' is under review. There are also significant variations in interpretation of existing rules between individual coroners and crematoria. As trusts will have their own policies with regard to dealing with the death of a patient, you are strongly advised to read them.

The Coroner's Officers must be informed of all reportable deaths. These are usually civilians employed by the local police, or police officers. They seldom have a medical background and this should be borne in mind when giving medical information, although their experience is usually sufficient for one not to be aware of this.

Cases requiring reporting

The cases requiring reporting are categorised in instructions to Registrars of Deaths but the cases you are likely to be involved with include the following.
○ Deaths in hospital:
  ‣ within 24 hours of admission
  ‣ during an operation
  ‣ before recovery from anaesthetic
  ‣ within 24 hours of leaving theatre
  ‣ where the conduct of a member of staff is called into question.
○ In addition, there are cases which you might experience in A&E and which usually result in an inquest. They are generally non-natural causes of death:
  ‣ cause unknown
  ‣ has occurred in suspicious circumstances
  ‣ due to violence or neglect

- due to an accident, whether at home, at work, or any other situation
- occurs in or shortly after prison or police custody
- alcoholic poisoning
- drugs or poisons
- abortion
- stillbirth if there is any reason to believe that the child was born alive
- industrial disease or industrial poisoning
- septicaemia associated with an injury or industrial disease
- possible homicide or manslaughter
- death due to trauma
- suspected suicide
- death not due to natural causes
- patient has not been seen in last illness (normally 14 days)
- sudden unexpected death including epilepsy or cot death.

Cases relating to violence or injury are still reportable even later, when death occurs less than a year and a day after the event causing the injury. An injury includes burns, choking, fractures (pathological fractures are usually excluded), foreign bodies, concussion, cuts, drowning, hyperthermia and hypothermia, sunstroke, lightning, electric shock, etc.

Unless it is clear that the death is due to a known natural cause it will normally be necessary for a post-mortem examination to be carried out. The permission of the relatives is not needed, but they of course must be informed and notified of the time and place unless this would unduly delay the examination. The relatives and other recognised persons are entitled to be represented at the post-mortem examination by a medical practitioner.

Action

Check out the written guidelines your hospital has for reporting cases to the coroner.

An inquest

Following a coroner's post-mortem an inquest may be held, the purpose of which will be to establish who died, when they died, where they died and how they died. The inquest is an inquiry into the causes of death. It is not an inquiry to determine blame. Your most likely appearance is in the coroner's court at an inquest. Some families may regard the inquest as an extension of the funeral and may find it a very distressing experience. For this reason alone it may be advisable to dress soberly and act appropriately and avoid using medical jargon or words not easily understood when answering any questions from the family.

When the coroner's office issues the request they are generally helpful and happy to informally liaise with the coroner and give information and assistance to the doctor preparing his report. Should the original records be released to the coroner it is advisable to make a complete copy.

Coroner's Courts Inquests are inquisitorial not adversarial, the coroner playing the inquiring role in that they conduct proceedings and ask most of the questions. They will examine and cross-examine witnesses under oath. Any lawyers attending on behalf of the estate or any next of kin of the deceased will be given the opportunity of asking the witnesses questions but will be pulled up if their questions turn to deal with the issue of blameworthiness rather than the cause of death.

The coroner usually sits alone, although a jury is required in cases of death occurring in prison or police custody or where it has resulted from an accident, poisoning or disease, notice of which is required to be given to a government department. Juries are also necessary in circumstances where the continuance of a possible recurrence might be prejudicial to the health or safety of the public. Unless there is an application for evidence to be heard in camera (i.e. a case involving the security services for example), an inquest takes place in open court. The inquests are often tape-recorded and evidence and any arguments are written down.

Various types of witnesses are called for facts such as evidence of identification, usually provided by a member of the family, although it could be the doctor or nurse or someone else that knew the deceased well. Mostly, the witnesses will be to facts, although the usual rules of evidence as regards hearsay do not apply and the coroner has the final say over what questions may or may not be asked. The coroner also determines what witnesses will be called and the order in which they will be called but any party has the right to ask the coroner to take evidence from witnesses. The coroner will usually call witnesses in such order as to give a clear account, in sequence, of the events leading up to the deceased's death. Where there is an individual who appears to be responsible for the death, he or she would normally be called last.

The witnesses are sworn or affirm and identify themselves. The coroner will usually lead the witnesses through their statements previously prepared and provided to the coroner usually via the Coroners Officer, who is usually a Police Officer. The coroner will usually confirm evidence of the witnesses, such as:
- relationship to or knowledge of the deceased
- the events leading up to or including the incident leading to the death
- the deceased's general state of health; this is more likely where the psychiatric nurse will be called to give evidence on behalf of the deceased who may have been a patient.

The coroner

A coroner is an independent judicial officer of the Crown whose duties are as assigned under the Statute of the Coroners' Act 1988. The coroner must be a registered medical practitioner, barrister or solicitor of a least five years standing and they investigate the circumstances of certain deaths. Each year in the UK about 180 000 cases are reported to a coroner, over half by doctors.

There will normally be guidelines written for your trust, particularly for dealing with cases which may have implications for the reputation of the hospital or the staff and especially in cases in which there may be media interest, although a coroner is not allowed to apportion blame for a death. At an inquest a coroner may allow questioning by lawyers representing the family of the deceased. Trusts normally provide appropriate managerial, legal and personal support. Common verdicts include accidental death, misadventure, suicide, industrial disease, natural causes, and an open verdict.

The coroner has the power to subpoena a witness and to impose a fine of up to £1000 or imprisonment for contempt of court for non-attendance. However, they are usually mindful of a doctor's other commitments and will often accept a written report from a doctor, such as the deceased's GP. If you are planning any leave in the period that may coincide with the inquest, it is strongly advised that you notify the coroner's office as soon as possible so that attempts can be made to avoid a clash. In cases where the medical issues are complex, it is possible that the coroner may ask for the opinion of an independent expert.

It is also worth noting that a coroner can accept so-called hearsay evidence of another person, unlike a criminal court. This usually takes the form of the results of tests, X-rays and biopsies by another doctor not present in the court.

Giving evidence

For the court's convenience and sometimes the convenience of the witnesses, medical experts might be allowed to give their evidence before the evidence as to facts. Careful preparation and familiarity with the events of the case are important. Witnesses are generally put at ease, and the procedure is more informal than other courts. Witnesses still take an oath or affirm. Each witness is taken through their statement by the coroner and questions asked where necessary. It might proceed something like the following.

o   Your name is (name)?
o   Your address is (address)?
o   You are a (type of doctor) doctor?
o   You are based at (name of hospital, etc)?
o   On (date) or during (dates) you interviewed and/or examined, counselled or treated (name of the deceased)?
o   You now produce (previous written report) your report on the deceased's condition and/or treatment.

Once the witnesses have given their evidence, the coroner will ask anyone present whether or not they would like to ask the witness questions. Family or their representatives can then ask questions. The witness could then be cross-examined by the deceased's' family lawyer with a view to obtaining further information regarding the death, particularly if the family are unhappy or angry. Defence organisations will often be prepared to give you advice if you are worried by the experience of appearing at an inquest.

The normal approach to dealing with legal decisions in English courts is by adversarial debate. Coroner's inquests are different. This is an inquiry, not adversarial, so coroners will not usually tolerate hostile questioning of witnesses. Where there is disagreement between witnesses the coroner will hear all evidence and the evidence thus presented enables the coroner to reach a verdict.

Solicitors may view an inquest as a preliminary investigation to a claim, but it is not for the coroner to apportion blame or deal with matters of negligence or civil liability. If your professional conduct or competence should be called into question you may seek an adjournment of the inquest from the coroner and contact your defence organisation for further advice. You are not obliged to answer questions that may incriminate you.

If there has been prior criticism of a doctor or you know that the family plan to be represented by a solicitor, often your defence organisation will instruct a solicitor on your behalf. This situation is rare.

Lawyers often advise witnesses to follow three 'golden rules'. They are:
○ dress up
○ speak up, then
○ shut up!

So, it is sensible to dress for the occasion, to take notes with you to refer to, having rehearsed them so that you can deliver your message with confidence, and, when you have said what you planned to say, sit down as soon as you have given simple answers to any questions. Do not dig a hole for yourself. If you do not know the answer, be honest and say so. Speculation or trying to be helpful is a pitfall to avoid at all costs. If you wish to refer to the records, ask to be allowed to do so.

In a trust it is usual for an individual to be designated the task of co-ordinating the gathering of information and providing this for the coroner. The report should be factual and accurate. You should refresh your memory as to the sequence of events using medical records, which are an essential part of the investigation. Avoid technical language and detailed explanation of complex procedures. Times of events should be given as precisely as possible. An account of the practitioner's personal involvement should be in sequence. Other staff should be identified so that their comments can be sought where necessary. If the deceased was a trust patient, the trust solicitor may attend on behalf of the hospital.

Summing up and conclusions

At the end of the hearing and after considering all the evidence the coroner will sum up if there is a jury directing them on points of law. This would happen if the death:
○ occurred in prison
○ occurred in police custody
○ was due to a notifiable disease
○ was due to an accident, or
○ occurred 'in circumstances the continuance or possible recurrence of which is prejudicial to the health or safety of the public or any section of the public'.

It is not common for the coroner to sit with a jury so if the coroner is sitting alone it is not necessary for them to sum up on the evidence although, in practice, the coroner may refer to it briefly. The coroner will then usually state in public the verdict they have reached.

The verdict will include the deceased's name, the injury or disease causing the death, the time, the place and circumstances in which the injury occurred, the determined cause of death and the registration particulars.

The coroners' rules allow no verdict to be framed in a way which appears to determine criminal or civil liability. Inevitably, the verdict which gives rise to most concern is lack of care. The court of appeal has recommended that this be replaced by 'to which neglect contributed'. The coroner is not permitted to apportion blame for the death.

The most common verdicts are:

- natural causes
- accidental death
- misadventure
- suicide
- industrial disease
- dependence on drugs
- non-dependent abuse of drugs
- killed himself or herself while the balance of the mind was disturbed
- attempted/self-induced abortion
- open verdict
- lawful killing
- unlawful killing
- stillbirth.

The words 'and that the cause of death was aggravated by a lack of care/self-neglect' may be added if appropriate. An open verdict may be returned where there is insufficient evidence to return any other suggested verdict.

The decision of the coroner can be subject to judicial review where the facts and evidence do not justify the verdict.

In Scotland there is no coroner's officer and a Fatal Accident Inquiry is heard by the Procurator Fiscal who investigates all sudden, suspicious, accidental, unexpected and unexplained deaths. The Procurator Fiscal should hold the inquiry before the Sheriff issues the final report (known as the 'Sheriff's Determination').

Witnesses will be paid their fees and reimbursed all reasonably incurred expenses immediately after the inquest. These fees are set by the Home Secretary and you are advised to contact the Clerk of the Court after the hearing to claim your fees.

Confidentiality

If a coroner asks for a statement or disclosure of the medical records, consent from the deceased's representative is not necessary, although you may wish to inform the family. If, however, information about living patients related to the deceased is requested you will need their consent.

The duty of confidentiality, however, does not end with a patient's death. After the inquest there may be questions from the press. It is acceptable and courteous to publicly convey sympathy to the family. It is not appropriate without consent of the family to volunteer further information. Never talk to the press without professional guidance. With regard to dealing with the media in a crisis remember the following.

○ Remain calm.
○ Think before you speak, preferably from a prepared statement.
○ Don't get drawn into any conversation.
○ Don't breach patient confidentiality.
○ Don't lose your cool.
○ Be reassured that even the media have to take account of guidelines and the laws of libel.
○ Call your defence society as early as possible and seek help.

For members of the MDU a 24-hour press office helpline (020 7202 1535 during office hours and 0800 716 646 out of hours) is available to assist its members with media inquiries in these circumstances.

You should go to the GMC website for further useful information on the following topics:

○ the duties of a doctor registered with the General Medical Council
○ patients' right to confidentiality
○ principles
○ protecting information
○ sharing information with patients
○ disclosing information about patients
○ circumstances where patients may give implied consent to disclosure
○ sharing information in the healthcare team or with others providing care
○ disclosing information for clinical audit
○ disclosures where express consent must be sought
○ disclosure in connection with judicial or other statutory proceedings
○ disclosures required by law
○ disclosures to the courts or in connection with litigation
○ disclosures to statutory regulatory bodies
○ disclosures in the public interest
○ disclosures to protect the patient or others
○ children and other patients who may lack competence to give consent
○ disclosures in relation to the treatment sought by children or others who lack capacity to give consent
○ disclosures where a patient may be a victim of neglect or abuse
○ disclosures after a patient's death.

Cremations

New cremation regulations came into force in January 2009, and introduced new forms for certification of cremation, replacing those that had been in force since 1930 and which were criticised in Dame Janet Smith's Third Report of the Shipman Inquiry in 2003. The Ministry of Justice has said that the regulations are an interim measure and that there are longer-term Department of Health plans to reform the entire death certification process.

Form Cremation 4 (Medical Certificate) essentially replaces Form B and form Cremation 5 (Confirmatory Medical Certificate) replaces Form C. The other key points are as follows.

Who can complete Cremation Certificates?

The doctor signing form Cremation 4 would be expected to have treated the deceased during the last illness and to have normally seen him or her within 14 days of death. The doctor who completes form Cremation 5 must have been registered as a medical practitioner for at least five years. They should not be a partner or colleague in the same practice or clinical team of the doctor who has completed form Cremation 4, nor can they be related to the deceased. Medical referees will need to be satisfied that the doctors who complete forms Cremation 4 and Cremation 5 are sufficiently independent of each other.

According to recent guidance from the RCGP and BMA on pandemic flu, during a flu pandemic, the government may announce a change to the regulations so that doctors who have not attended the patient may be allowed to complete a streamlined form Cremation 4, while the requirement for form Cremation 5 could be suspended, removing the need for a second doctor to confirm information.

The new cremation forms

While the new forms do not differ significantly from the old forms, the doctor responsible for filling in form Cremation 5 is required to thoroughly check both forms and to query any inconsistencies. However, there are some aspects of the guidance which may cause confusion and there is guidance on this at the MDU website www.the-mdu.com (search for 'new cremation rules'). In the summary that guidance states: 'It is expected that at least one of questions 2 to 5 of form Cremation 5 will be answered in the affirmative.' However, in the section addressing requirements for form Cremation 5, it says: 'We consider that, with the exception of questions 6 and 7, you should answer in the affirmative all the questions in Part 2 in all but the most extreme circumstances' (paragraph 30, p. 11).

The MDU sought clarification from the Coroners' Unit at the Ministry of Justice on this point. They will be amending their guidance in due course, but in the meantime have asked us to make clear that doctors only need to answer yes to one question on form Cremation 5.

Paragraph 30 also states that: 'Question 2 should be answered in the affirmative only if you have seen and questioned a medical practitioner other than the form Cremation [4] doctor'. However, the form itself refers only to having questioned another medical practitioner and does not suggest that this must be face to face. The MDU believes that it will be sufficient for doctors to have spoken to another medical practitioner by telephone, although they will be expected to indicate whether they spoke to them in person or by telephone.

Cause of death

The guidance makes clear that the cause of death should normally be that set out on the medical certificate of the cause of death sent to the Registrar of Deaths. However, it says that medical referees are likely to reject forms without a proper cause of death. For example, the guidance says that 'multi-organ failure' and 'heart attack' are unacceptable, while 'old age' alone is 'unlikely to be acceptable'.

New rights for families of the deceased

Under the Cremation Regulations 2008 patients' relatives have the right to inspect the medical forms about the death. Inspection of the forms should take place before the cremation is authorised by the medical referee. This might occur if a relative had doubts or was surprised that the death occurred. They can also nominate someone else to inspect the forms on their behalf.

If they have serious concerns about the death and believe a coroner should investigate the case, they may contact the coroner's office. The forms are normally available for inspection at the crematorium office for up to 48 hours after the relatives are informed that they have been received there. The medical referee may be able to give advice on the cause of death, but may charge a fee for this service.

Given that 'some of the information which is requested by the forms may have been given to the deceased in confidence', it advises that in such cases, doctors 'may give the information to the medical referee on a separate sheet of paper attached to the form explaining your reasons for this and that the information should not be disclosed'.

It is worth noting that a pacemaker can explode on cremation, causing damage to the crematorium equipment and therefore a doctor signing Cremation 4 (Medical Certificate) must state that any pacemaker has been removed; the crematorium referee will check this confirmation before authorising the cremation.

Guidance for doctors is available from the Home Office and can be downloaded from their website (www.dh.gov.uk/cmo), following links to 'cremation'. The guidance is part of a drive to tighten the authorisation procedures following the Shipman Inquiry. Guidance can also be obtained at your medical protection society, such as MDU or MPS and you can also find lots of information at their websites (www.themdu.com and www.medicalprotection.org/uk). And of course on www.doctors.net.uk you'll find all sorts of advice and tales of experiences about the subject.

Action

If you have time, why not go and see an inquest? A call to the Coroners Office will tell you when the next cases are scheduled. You may find it helpful to refer to the following for more information.

Resources

Books

Burton J, Rutty G. *The Hospital Autopsy*. 3rd ed. London: Hodder Arnold; 2009.

Levine M, Pyke J. *Levine on Coroners' Courts*. London: Sweet & Maxwell; 1998.

Online with full text

McDermott MB. Obtaining consent for autopsy. *BMJ*. 2003; **327**: 804–6. Available online at www.bmj.com/cgi/content/extract/327/7418/804

Ministry of Justice. *Cremation Regulations 2008: guidance for doctors*. Ministry of Justice; 2008. Available online at www.justice.gov.uk/about/docs/cremation-doctors-guidance.pdf

O'Grady G. Death of the teaching autopsy. *BMJ*. 2003; **327**: 802–3. Available online at www.bmj.com/cgi/content/extract/327/7418/802

RCGP, BMA. *Preparing for Pandemic Influenza*. RCGP and BMA; December 2008 (published January 2009). Available online at www.rcgp.org.uk/pdf/gp_guidance.pdf

Report of the Joint Working Party of the Royal College of Pathologists, the Royal College of Physicians of London and the Royal College of Surgeons of England. *The Autopsy and Audit*. RCPath, RCP and RCS; 1991. Available online at Resuscitation Council website www.resus.org.uk.

Underwood J. Commentary: resuscitating the teaching autopsy. *BMJ*. 2003; **327**: 803–4. Available online at www.bmj.com/cgi/content/extract/327/7418/803

Other online sources

○ Royal College of Pathologists, www.rcpath.org.
○ Home Office, www.homeoffice.gov.uk.
○ The Shipman Inquiry, www.the-shipman-inquiry.org.uk.
○ Department of Health, www.dh.gov.uk.
○ King's College, London has some useful information on Coroner's Rules, www.kcl.ac.uk.
○ The Coroners' Society of England and Wales, www.coroner.org.uk.
○ Cremation Society of Great Britain: Arrangement of Regulations, www.srgw.demon.co.uk/CremSoc/.
○ For links to the Pathology Specialties Forum and Medico-Legal Forum, www.doctors.net.uk.

When things go wrong

The National Patient Safety Agency guidelines, *Being Open*, were published in November 2009 (NPSA 2009), and urge 'effective communication' with patients, their families and carers. It states that the NHS should be open with patients when things go wrong – including being ready to say sorry, according to guidelines.

It says that 'Evidence from other countries shows that by following the principles of *Being Open*, formal complaints and litigation claims can also be reduced.' Certainly the guidelines are backed by RCOG, RCPsy, RCN. A spokesman for the MDU said that, 'Doctors have an ethical obligation to offer an apology and an explanation if something has gone wrong and there is no legal reason not to do so.' NHS Medical

Director Professor Sir Bruce Keogh said: 'Being open with patients should anything go wrong with their healthcare is the right thing to do.'

The guidance includes recommendations and actions for improving the effectiveness of *Being Open* for boards, clinicians, PALS and other healthcare professionals. For further information go to the NPSA website at www.nrls.npsa.nhs.uk/resources/?entryid45=65077 where you can download the three documents; *Being Open – communicating patient safety incidents with patients, their families and carers, Being Open – supporting information*, and *Being Open – framework*.

Complaints

Sometimes things do go wrong and result in complaints. Complaints fall into three main areas.

○ Complaints, whether clinical or non-clinical, may be made against you or the hospital by dissatisfied patients and relatives with whom you have direct contact.
○ Complaints about the whole team, medical outcomes, administrative and support service and the hospital generally. These can be made by patients and relatives or organisations representing patients' interests.
○ Internal employee complaints made against the hospital.

In the next section I will deal mainly with those instances where you are faced with a patient bringing a complaint. The following section outlines the procedures for dealing with more formal complaints. Employment complaints are normally the subject of internal trust procedures and are monitored by the personnel department. If you do become involved in a complaint related to employment, I suggest you contact the local BMA office and seek the advice of the Industrial Relations Officer.

Dealing with an informal patient complaint

Patients initially have three options for complaining or obtaining advice on complaints.

○ The liaison service (PALS) staff or complaints manager at the NHS trust hospital or primary care trust involved in the complaint. They may be able to resolve the problem on the spot or will provide details of how to complain.
○ NHS Direct, Tel: 0845 4647.
○ The Independent Complaints Advocacy Service (ICAS).

Complaints are usually due to one or more of the following:
○ actual or perceived failure of doctor to deliver expected standard of care
○ unrealistic expectation of patient or relatives
○ failure of communication.

A complaint is not a claim but it could become one. It is important that it is be handled well. Usually, this means a prompt explanation to any patient or their relative involved in any event that has given rise to the complaint. Minor criticism should be dealt with by conciliation not confrontation. Deal with the situation sympathetically. An apology can be given, as an apology is not an admission of legal liability.

If you find yourself first in line when a patient or relative complains it is helpful to remember that the complainant is usually angry, so:

o try to be on a level with the other person; if you are looking down on them they may feel more threatened

o allow them plenty of personal space and do not get too close, this also may make them feel threatened

o acknowledge their feelings by an empathic statement; the other person now understands that you appreciate their position and they no longer have to prove their anger

o indicate that you are listening by reflective listening, repeating back a summary of what is being said

o avoid questioning an angry person

o if you are in a closed space or room, check that you are well positioned for leaving quickly, or at least ensure that a large piece of furniture separates you from the complainant!

Use simple assertiveness techniques (*see* Chapter 2 on assertiveness) such as the 'broken record' to express yourself calmly and persistently as the angry person often leaps from topic to topic.

They may use criticism as a weapon and again the 'broken record' technique is useful. It can be helpful to use another assertiveness technique called 'fogging'. This is simply a method of taking the wind out of your critic's sails by saying that there may be some truth in what they saying or agreeing in principle with them.

Safety considerations

In 2005 the Healthcare Commission reported that a quarter of NHS staff reported abuse or harassment by patients in the previous year, with 14% being physically attacked. Despite claims of a 'zero tolerance' approach to violence against staff, the most recent figures from 2002–3 found that 116 000 incidents of verbal and physical abuse had been reported by NHS staff. The number of successful prosecutions against people who assaulted NHS staff rose sharply in the following year, according to statistics from the Department of Health that show that in 2004–5 there were 759 successful prosecutions, compared to 51 in the previous year.

Employers are responsible for ensuring that employees are kept safe at work and the Health and Safety Act (1974) and ensuing amendments emphasises the need for assessment of risks and adequate training. There is also a responsibility on the employee to take reasonable steps to safeguard their own safety and health at work. The following pointers may be useful.

o There should be security systems in place.

o Layout of the room should be considered, doors opening outwards, observation panels and removal of potential missiles.

o There should be protocols for seeing patients with another member of staff nearby.

○ CCTV, panic buttons and personal alarms may be necessary.
○ Staff should be trained in personal safety and breakaway techniques.
○ It is always important to review a patient's history for previous violence, mental health problems and history of alcohol or drug abuse.
○ For any home visits there must be a protocol for letting people know where you are and your expected return time.

Personal safety

○ Use your work address in the Medical Directory.
○ Use an ex-directory home telephone number.
○ Be aware of the dangers of ties and scarves when seeing at-risk patients.
○ Be aware of body language signs.
○ Avoid prolonged eye contact.
○ Position yourself in a room nearest the door and if necessary leave the door open.
○ Know about the safety procedures in your unit and the position of panic buttons.

During an interview about a complaint or even during a consultation be aware of the possible signs of pending violence:
○ raised tone of voice
○ raised volume of voice
○ red face
○ clenched fists
○ pointing fingers
○ invasion of personal space
○ verbal threats
○ refusal to communicate
○ restlessness
○ pacing about.

Use your communication skills to take the heat out of the situation once you see signs of impending violence. Once things have progressed beyond a certain point this may be futile and at this stage you should leave the situation as soon as possible. However, before you have made that decision you could try:
○ active listening with open questions
○ reassurance and acknowledgement of grievances
○ good but not persistent and prolonged eye contact, which might be considered threatening
○ keeping your distance, but away from corners where you could be trapped
○ asking for any weapons to be put down rather than handed over
○ using the panic button or calling for help
○ leaving the room and getting assistance from security or police.

If an incident occurs, it has further implications for the individuals concerned and other members of staff, so the following will be required:

o fill out an incident report form
o discuss it with colleagues
o document it in patient's notes so that subsequent staff are aware of the history
o consider pressing charges
o in general practice, consider removing patient from list
o seek counselling if required
o consider the Criminal Injuries Compensation Authority or NHS Injury Benefit Scheme
o consider how you handled the situation and whether you need further training.

When a patient assaults a doctor they forego a degree of their right to confidentiality. While reporting the incident to the police, the doctor can only provide essential details but no clinical details. Under certain circumstances, however, clinical details may be disclosed if the withholding of such information places the patient or others at risk of serious harm or death. If you are attacked, you can also discuss these issues with your defence organisation.

According to the *Health Service Journal* (6 November 2008), more than 55 000 physical assaults were reported against NHS staff in England in 2007/8. Figures collated by the NHS Security Management Service (NHS SMS) reveal that 55 993 attacks were reported in 2007/8, a rise of 284 from the previous year. There were 759 successful prosecutions in England in 2004/5 compared to 51 in 2002/3. NHS Security Management Service data showed there were 58 695 physical assaults against NHS staff in England in 2005/6, and all assaults against staff working in NHS hospitals rose. The NHS SMS has launched a comprehensive strategy to better protect staff and property in the NHS, with a particular emphasis on tackling violence. *See* www.nhsbsa. nhs.uk/SecurityManagement.aspx, where you will find more detailed guidance and information on this subject and what the NHS is doing to try to tackle the problem.

The NHS Security Management Service was established in 2003, creating the NHS Counter Fraud and Security Management Service, of which the latter is responsible for the security of NHS staff and property in England, the first time a dedicated organisation has had such a remit. This includes:

o protecting NHS staff from violence and abuse
o taking appropriate action against those who abuse, or attempt to abuse, NHS staff
o helping to ensure the security of property, facilities, equipment and other resources, such as drugs.

All NHS health bodies have to nominate a director at board level to take responsibility for security management, ensuring that security of NHS staff and property is considered at the highest levels. More serious complaints should be reported and handled by formal procedures as they may lead to a claim for compensation. These should be referred to a person of sufficient seniority for them to deal with the situation as required. Most trusts have well-documented procedures for handling complaints and these should always be followed.

NHS complaints procedure

If a patient is unhappy with their treatment or the service they have received from the NHS they are entitled to make a complaint, have it considered, and receive a response from the NHS organisation or primary care practitioner concerned. Your trust is certain to have written guidelines on its complaints procedure. A new NHS and social care complaints procedure was introduced in England in April 2009, the key points of which are as follows. There are some differences in the way the procedures in Scotland, Wales and Northern Ireland operate and these are indicated towards the end of the chapter.

The two-stage procedure

One of the more significant changes is that the procedure now has just two stages – local resolution and, for complainants who remain dissatisfied, referral to the Health Service Ombudsman. The second stage of the old complaints procedure, an independent review by the Healthcare Commission, no longer exists.

Most complaints seem to be resolved quickly and efficiently at local resolution. Complainants who are not satisfied with a response provided at local resolution may refer the matter to the Ombudsman, as can doctors who are unhappy with the first stage; for example, if they do not agree with a response provided on their behalf by a PCT.

Under these new regulations, patients can choose whether to complain to the organisation providing care (hospital or GP surgery) or to the commissioning body (usually the PCT). Where a complaint is directed to the PCT and the PCT considers it more appropriate for the provider to respond, the complaint can be passed to the provider so long as the patient consents to this. However, if a complaint handled by a GP or the practice is not resolved satisfactorily at the local level, the regulations do not allow the complainant to seek a review from the PCT. If the complainant then wants to pursue the complaint further, it must be referred to the Ombudsman.

Every NHS organisation has a complaints procedure. You ought to find out about it because a patient could ask. There is usually information on a hospital or trust's website, and you could refer any inquiry to the complaints department for more information. The NHS Constitution gives everyone the right to make a complaint and to:

- have a complaint dealt with efficiently and have it properly investigated
- know the outcome of any investigation into the complaint
- take your complaint to the independent Parliamentary and Health Service Ombudsman if you are not satisfied with the way the NHS has dealt with your complaint
- make a claim for judicial review if you think you have been directly affected by an unlawful act or decision of an NHS body
- receive compensation where you have been harmed.

Complainants are normally current or former patients or nominated representatives, which can include a solicitor or a patient's elected representative, for example an MP. If someone other than the patient makes a complaint, it is important to ensure they have authority to do so. If a patient lacks capacity to make decisions for themselves, the representative must be able to demonstrate sufficient interest in their welfare and be an appropriate person to act on their behalf. Patients over the age of 16 whose mental capacity is unimpaired should normally complain themselves. Children under the age of 16 who are able to do so may make their own complaint.

Responsible bodies (PCTs, hospital trusts, primary care providers and other organisations providing NHS services) are required to have a 'responsible person' who will usually be the most senior person in the organisation, such as a chief executive in a trust, or a senior partner in primary care. The responsible person must ensure the organisation complies with the complaints regulations and that any actions identified as necessary during the investigation of a complaint are taken. The responsible person, or someone authorised to act on their behalf, must 'sign off' all complaint responses and, even if the responsible person delegates this responsibility, he or she still remains accountable under the regulations. Responsible bodies must have a 'complaints manager' who is readily accessible to the public. The complaints manager co-ordinates the investigation of, and responses to, complaints as well as co-ordinating other requirements on the monitoring and reporting of complaints. The complaints manager may, if authorised, sign responses on behalf of the responsible person.

The regulations require all responsible bodies to make arrangements for dealing with complaints to ensure:
- complaints are dealt with efficiently
- complaints are properly investigated
- complainants are treated with respect and courtesy
- complainants receive, so far as is reasonably practical, assistance to enable them to understand the procedure in relation to complaints or advice on where they may obtain such assistance
- complainants receive a timely and appropriate response
- complainants are told the outcome of the investigation of their complaint; and action is taken if necessary in the light of the outcome of the complaint.

The complaint should be made within 12 months from the date on which the matter occurred, or from when the matter came to the attention of the complainant. The regulations, however, allow a responsible body to consider complaints outside that limit. An extension might be possible, for example, in situations where it would have been difficult to complain earlier because of grief or trauma.

The previous regulations required a full, detailed and positive response to be provided within 10 working days of receipt in primary care, and 20 days in secondary care. These rather restrictive limits have been removed in the new procedures in order to provide ample opportunity for an appropriate level of investigation to take place at the local resolution stage. The new regulations do not set timescales, but they do require a timely and appropriate response.

The response to a complaint
- The regulations require complaints (other than oral complaints that can be resolved in one working day) to be acknowledged within three working days.

○ The complaints manager must make a written record of the date on which a complaint was received and needs to provide the complainant with a written record of the complaint, even if it was made verbally or electronically.

○ The complainant should be offered the opportunity to discuss an agreed approach to the complaint, either by telephone or in person. The complainant should then be informed how the complaint is to be handled; for example, given details of how it is to be investigated, and of the expected timescales for a response.

○ If a response is not provided within six months from the date the complaint was made, or a later date if one was agreed with the complainant, the complaints manager must write to the complainant and explain the delay.

○ If it is possible to resolve a simple oral complaint within 24 hours and the patient is happy with the response, the regulations do not require a formal written response, though that does not prevent confirmation of the discussion in writing if appropriate.

○ A note of the oral complaint, and the response to it, should be made and kept in a complaint file. It does not need to be included in the annual report on complaints, as it does not fall within the regulations. However, this does not prevent it being considered under local clinical governance procedures.

○ The regulations require the response to contain an explanation of how the complaint was investigated and details of conclusions reached. It should identify any matters that need remedial action and explain whether such action is planned or has already taken place.

○ The report should explain the complainant's right to take the matter to the Ombudsman within 12 months if dissatisfied with the response.

Complaints are recorded and monitored and an annual report prepared, which has to be available to anyone who asks to see it, and sent to the PCT by primary care providers. The complaints record should include the subject matter of the complaint, the outcome and any lessons that have been learned. The annual report should give details of the complaints received and identify those considered to be 'well-founded'. It should also contain details of complaints referred to the Ombudsman and any lessons learnt, particularly if there are any patterns of complaints that developed in the reporting period.

If you have any concerns with complaints you should always contact your defence organisation for advice.

There is help available for complainants from the Patient Advice or Liaison Service (PALS) for which officers are available in all hospitals. They can offer confidential advice, support and information on health-related matters to patients, their families and their carers. They can also contact a local PALS office by accessing the Office Directory at PALS online at www.pals.nhs.uk/officemapsearch.aspx. The other source of help is The Independent Complaints Advocacy Service (ICAS), a national service that supports people who wish to make a complaint about their NHS care or treatment. They can be contacted through a local ICAS office in about 11 offices spread around the country.

Failing that, the local Citizens Advice Bureau can be a great source for advice and support for those wanting to complain about the NHS. They can be found at local Citizens Advice Bureau on the bureau's website or in a local telephone directory. And finally NHS Direct can advise on NHS complaints.

Legislation and guidance relating to the new NHS complaints procedure is available to download at www.dh.gov.uk/en/Managingyourorganisation/Legalandcontractual/Complaintspolicy/NHScomplaintsprocedure/DH_376. There is also information on how to complain for members of the public as well as on the process of reform and training for NHS staff.

All NHS trusts and health authorities have to provide information to all patients about their right to complain, and provide advice about how to use the complaints procedure, and what help is available to complainants.

Health Service Commissioner (Ombudsman)

Complainants who remain dissatisfied after the NHS complaints procedure has been completed may ask the Health Service Commissioner (Ombudsman) to investigate their case. The Ombudsman is completely independent of the NHS and of the government, and can consider complaints about most aspects of NHS services and treatment. However, they are not obliged to investigate every complaint put to them.

The Health Service Commissioner has the power to investigate written complaints from the public about the provision of services or maladministration. The commission has the power to examine internal papers and clinical records. Any doctor faced with a request to give a report should take advice.

The Health Service Ombudsman can only help you if the complaint is about NHS or NHS-funded healthcare in England. Complaints about healthcare in Scotland, Wales and Northern Ireland have to be made to the appropriate Ombudsman. It is also possible to contact the local ICAS that supports patients and their carers who wish to pursue a complaint about any NHS treatment or care. The Ombudsman cannot look into complaints about privately funded healthcare. There is no independent complaint handler for complaints about private healthcare. Patients unhappy about treatment or service received from a private healthcare provider have to complain to them directly.

Further information about the Ombudsman can be seen at www.ombudsman.org.uk.

Roles of parties to a complaint

There may be any number of parties involved in a complaint. The following is a summary of those who might be involved and some aspects of their roles.

Patient's advocate

If the complainant is not the patient it is important to be clear just what the nature of the complaint is and the complainant's perspective: is the complainant acting on behalf of the patient and, if so, do they have the authority of the patient to do so?

Patient's family or carers

It should be established whether the complainant is acting on behalf of a wider group, or drawing upon a wider knowledge base than is immediately obvious.

Convenor

The convenor is a non-executive director appointed by the board to manage the independent review panel process. Where a complaint relates in whole or in part to action taken in exercising clinical judgement, the convenor must take appropriate clinical advice.

Independent Complaints Advocacy Service

Set up in September 2003, the Independent Complaints Advocacy Service can help patients to make their complaint or give help with making a complaint. Trained advocates, also known as caseworkers, with knowledge of the NHS complaints procedure, help clients to understand whether they wish to pursue a complaint and, where needed, provide support to clients to do so. This support may range from helping with initial preparation in ordering their thoughts and thinking about what a good resolution would look like, through to attendance at resolution meetings, and helping with correspondence.

Four voluntary sector organisations deliver ICAS: Citizens Advice Bureau (CAB), the Carers' Federation, PohWER and South East Advocacy Projects (SEAP). The four providers took over cases from the old Community Health Councils (CHCs).

For more information look at their websites or go to www.dh.gov.uk/change agentteam.

Healthcare professionals

A complaint can harm a professional's career, especially if poorly handled. To ensure they do not feel excluded from the process they normally draft the response that will go to the complainant. If an apology is required, this can be the clinician's own letter with a follow-up by the chief executive, thus ensuring compliance with the regulations.

Professional bodies

Allowances are made in the planning for the involvement of a professional's representative body. The representative body can also provide independent support to a professional.

Trade unions

Trade unions or other staff bodies will be interested in the complaints procedure and likely to play an active part in supporting its members.

The media

The NHS is a popular topic for both local and national media. The episode may come under media scrutiny. Some letters may appear in the press if the complainant is unhappy.

The board

Complaints have to be reported to the board quarterly. The board has to produce an annual report on complaints handling and circulate it widely.

Health Service Commissioner (Ombudsman)

If a complainant is not successful in getting an independent review panel established, or is unhappy with the outcome of the panel, he or she can approach the Ombudsman.

Action for Victims of Medical Accidents

AVMA can provide patients or relatives with information about how to proceed with a complaint.

NHS complaints procedure in Scotland

The complaints procedure was amended in 2005 and a helpful guide to the new procedures, *Can I Help You?*, is available from www.show.scot.nhs.uk. One of the principles of the complaints procedure is to ensure clear lines of accountability for complaints management and integration into the organisation's clinical governance and quality improvement arrangements. In other words, it is a system designed for reviewing and learning from complaints. Complainants have to be informed of any action taken as a result of a complaint to prevent a recurrence of the same problem. The procedure has two stages: local resolution as a first stage; and patients who remain dissatisfied can complain direct to the Scottish Public Services Ombudsman.

A patient, former patient or their agent may make complaints. Where the patient is a child, the parent, guardian or person who has care of the child (e.g. the local authority) can make the complaint. If the patient is an adult who is incapable of making a complaint, a relative or 'other adult person who has an interest in their welfare' may complain. For deceased patients, a relative or other adult who had an interest in the patient's welfare may make a complaint. Bear in mind the importance of patient confidentiality, especially if the patient is not making the complaint, is a child or lacks capacity. If patients are deceased, the duty of confidence extends after death. If in any doubt, members should seek advice from their defence organisation.

There is a time limit of six months from the event that is the subject of the complaint, or six months from the patient becoming aware of the subject of the complaint provided this is not later than 12 months after the event. A complainant who believes a doctor's refusal to respond to a complaint is unreasonable may complain to the Ombudsman or the GMC.

Complaints must be acknowledged within three working days and a response should be provided within 20 working days (hospitals) and 10 working days (GPs), or as soon as is reasonably practicable. A timely response is more likely to resolve the complaint. If you cannot respond within the time limit, inform the complainant, give reasons for the delay and tell them when they may expect a response. *Can I Help You?* suggests the investigation should not normally take longer than 40 working days for hospitals or 20 working days for GPs, other than in exceptional circumstances. For advice on a written response you ought to consult your defence organisation, although many have written advice on writing a response to a complaint.

Hospital complaints 'may be investigated by the complaints officer in any manner which appears appropriate'. This may include offering the complainant a meeting with senior staff or a conciliation process. Any meetings or discussions should be documented carefully and a letter sent to the complainant setting out any agreements reached or further action to be taken. *Can I Help You?* advises that complaints records should usually be kept separate from health records. The guidance makes it clear that, for clinical complaints, the draft findings and response must be shown to the clinicians involved to ensure factual accuracy, before it is sent to the complainant. Given the importance of learning from complaints, and their use in appraisal, it is vital that clinicians are able to take part in the resolution of complaints about care they provide.

Health boards are required to provide conciliation services for complaints about GPs (at the request of the patient or the GP) where:

○ a person wishes to complain and, in the opinion of the health board, it would be unreasonable for the person to complain directly to the GP
○ a complaint is already being investigated by the GP
○ the practice-based complaints procedure has been completed and the complainant remains unsatisfied.

Both parties must agree to conciliation. The conciliator may adopt whatever procedures they consider appropriate.

The Scottish Public Services Ombudsman Act 2002 set up a single office to deal with complaints about a number of bodies, including the Scottish Executive and the health service (*see* www.scottishombudsman.org.uk). The Ombudsman's office usually only considers complaints that have been addressed fully by the complaints procedures of the body concerned, though there is the power to waive this requirement.

Possible outcomes from an Ombudsman investigation include:

○ an apology or explanation
○ practical action to mitigate any injustice
○ reimbursement of any actual losses/costs necessarily incurred
○ a modest payment in recognition of time and trouble
○ exceptionally, asking the authority complained about to propose appropriate action
○ recommending changes to procedure or policy
○ recommending staff guidance or training.

Compensation should only be paid if negligence has been proven. It has no part in the complaints procedure. You should seek the advice of your defence organisation when the question of any payment to the complainant might arise.

NHS complaints procedure in Wales

Complaints in the NHS is a guide to handling complaints in Wales that provides comprehensive details on how the NHS expects hospitals and GPs to manage patient complaints. The following key points are taken from that guidance.

The procedure in Wales is split into three stages.

1   Local resolution – by the hospital or practice.
2   Independent review – by the Independent Review Secretariat, separate from the NHS.
3   Pubic Services Ombudsman for Wales.

Anyone can complain who has used NHS services or facilities, or a relative or friend can on behalf of a patient. However, the patient must give written authority if the response might include personal information.

If a patient has died, the GP or hospital should proceed with an investigation. If the patient lacks capacity, the Mental Capacity Act 2005 provides for a person to be given lasting powers of attorney and if this extends to welfare decisions, that person would be able to make a complaint on behalf of someone lacking capacity. Otherwise, if the complainant is not the patient's next of kin, the patient's relatives need to be consulted, and their views considered. If the next of kin refuses to authorise an investigation, the guidance suggests it may be possible to respond generally, without breaching confidentiality, but members are advised to consult their defence organisation.

Only a child's parents or those with legal responsibility can bring complaints against a GP on behalf of a child under 16. However, if services are provided by a trust, local health board or independent provider, a Gillick competent child under 16 may complain on their own behalf.

As elsewhere in the UK, there is a period for making a complaint of six months from the event or within six months from the patient becoming aware of the subject of the complaint, provided this is not later than 12 months after the event. These guidelines operate flexibly: complaints would be accepted where it would be unreasonable for the patient to have complained earlier and it is still possible to investigate the facts. There may be many reasons why patients cannot bring their complaint within these timescales and dealing with the complaint, even some time after the event, may help to resolve a patient's concerns.

Local resolution

Complaints are first addressed locally within the GP practice or hospital. Often speed, sympathy and a willingness to listen and explain are all that are necessary to resolve concerns. Hospitals and practices should have a complaints manager who is responsible for the operation of the local resolution procedures, ensuring that the complaint is dealt with appropriately. Complaints need to be acknowledged within two working days.

Local resolution allows for a range of different options for responding to a complaint, which may include:
o   inviting the complainant to meet staff, practitioners and clinicians to discuss their concerns further (the complainant can bring a supporter, who may be legally qualified but not acting in a legal capacity)
o   arranging a second opinion on clinical issues
o   offering independent facilitation or mediation.

Once the investigation is complete, a full response has to be sent to the complainant within 20 working days. If it is not possible to complete the investigation within 20 days, complainants should be informed of the reason for the delay and told when they can expect to receive a reply. For advice on providing a written response you need to consult your defence organisation.

All Welsh GPs are required by their contract to have a practice-based system for handling complaints, complying with national criteria and guidance. Practices must co-operate with the NHS complaints procedure (and with the local health board), including independent review. For GPs, the local disciplinary procedure cannot be considered until the complaints procedure, including independent review, is exhausted.

Independent review

Complainants who are dissatisfied with local resolution may then request an independent review from the Independent Review Secretariat. This can be done orally or in writing within 28 days of being informed of the outcome of local resolution and complainants should be informed of this right in the full response.

The complainant or someone who has the patient's written permission must make the request for independent review. When the Secretariat receives such a request it sends a written acknowledgement of the request within two working days. It also informs the doctor and anyone else mentioned in the complaint that it has received a request for review.

The Secretariat then appoints an independent reviewer and lay adviser to consider the complaint. The reviewer and adviser are both independent laypeople appointed by and accountable to the Welsh Assembly. For clinical complaints, the Secretariat will also appoint a clinical adviser from the same profession or specialty as the doctor. The reviewer is responsible for deciding which course of action to take. They may:
o refer the case, or part of the case, back to local resolution, recommending actions that might resolve the complaint
o decide to set up a panel to investigate the complaint further
o recommend a more appropriate course of action outside the NHS complaints procedure
o decide to take no further action because local resolution has been carried out satisfactorily and achieved everything possible.

The reviewer then gives the complainant full reasons for the decision and advises them of their right to complain to the Ombudsman if they remain dissatisfied.

Public Services Ombudsman for Wales

If the complainant is unhappy with the outcome of independent review, or has not sought independent review, they can write to the Ombudsman and ask for a further investigation. Complainants need to provide reasons why they are still dissatisfied and feel that they have suffered hardship or injustice.

Practitioners and their staff may also complain to the Ombudsman about the local health board or NHS trust if they feel that they have been treated unfairly by the administration of the complaints process.

The Ombudsman will not accept a complaint older than 12 months unless there is a good reason why the complaint could not have been made earlier. The Ombudsman has no power to enforce recommendations or impose sanctions. Where the Ombudsman investigates a complaint, this will be reported in regular reports to the National Assembly of Wales.

NHS complaints procedure in Northern Ireland

Again it is a two-stage procedure that aims to obtain an explanation for what happened, an apology or other statement of regret and steps to review procedures to avoid such incidents in future. It does not offer financial compensation (although in some circumstances NHS bodies will agree to an ex-gratia payment for relatively small sums). Nor does it address issues of staff discipline, such as sacking staff or striking off a practitioner (although disciplinary action may result as a consequence of information obtained through complaints investigations). Nor does it address private treatment unless financed by the NHS.

A complaint has to be made no later than 12 months after the event or from the date the patient first became aware of the issues in question, although there is discretion to consider complaints outside this limit. A complaint can be made verbally, in writing or electronically. Where a complaint is made orally, the healthcare provider to whom the complaint is being made must make a written copy of the complaint and provide a copy of the written record to the complainant. It can be made to the hospital, practice or PCT.

The first stage is local resolution, where the NHS body or practice is required to investigate and respond to the complaint and provide an acknowledgement of the complaint no later than three working days after it has been received. The complainant should also:

o be offered the opportunity to discuss the complaint
o be advised of the way in which the complaint will be investigated
o be advised of the time within which the investigation of the complaint is likely to be completed
o when they are likely to receive the response and conclusion to the complaint and if there is likely to be a delay in the investigation and response, they should be notified in writing and given an explanation.

As part of the investigation, complainants may be invited to meetings, although often they may not want to see staff members who have been involved in the incident. In some cases complainants may be disappointed to find the staff involved are not available. After any such meeting, if the NHS organisation considers that the matter has been adequately addressed, they send a written response concluding the local resolution stage of the complaints procedure. This should also tell a patient what to do next if they are not satisfied. If a complainant commences legal action or says that this is their definite intention, the NHS complaints procedure can be brought to a close. If they are not satisfied with the response, they have the right to request an Independent Review.

The request for an Independent Review has to be made within 28 calendar days of the care provider's written response to the complaint. In Northern Ireland the complaints convenor at the local Health and Social Services Board considers requests for Independent Review and has the power to decide what happens next. The convenor/ reviewer tries to make a decision about convening a panel within 20 days for NHS trusts or 10 days for Family Health Service Complaints.

The options open to the convenor/reviewer are:

○ refer the complaint back for further investigation under the local resolution stage
○ recommend no further action if they feel that the complaint has been fully considered, but they must give reasons for this and inform of the right to complain to the Ombudsman
○ agree to set up an Independent Review panel.

The report will be sent to the chief executive of the body involved and also interested parties such as the staff involved. The chief executive then writes to the complainant within 20 working days to say what action is being taken in relation to the report. If the complainant is unhappy with the Independent Review report, they can complain to the Ombudsman. For those who require more information see the website at www. ni-ombudsman.org.uk/whatdo.htm.

Action

Look at the summary document of your trust's complaints procedure.

Related reading

AVMA website at www.avma.org.uk

Aylin P, Shivani T, Bottle A and Jarman B. How often are adverse events reported in English hospital statistics? *BMJ*. 2004; **329**(7462): 369.

Baile WF, Buckman R, Lenzi R *et al*. SPIKES: a six-step protocol for delivering bad news: application to the patient with cancer. *Oncologist*. 2000; **5**(4): 302–11.

BBC News and Information. Children 'must learn about death'. May 2004. See http://news. bbc.co.uk/2/hi/uk_news/education/3682381.stm

BMA. *Advance Statements about Medical Treatment*. London: British Medical Association; 1995.

BMA Medical Ethics Department at www.bma.org.uk

BMA, Resuscitation Council. *Decision Relating to Cardiopulmonary Resuscitation*. RCN; 2001.

Buckman R. *How to Break Bad News: a guide for health care professionals*. Baltimore, MD: Johns Hopkins University Press; 1992.

Burton J, Rutty G. *The Hospital Autopsy*. 3rd ed. London: Hodder Arnold; 2009.

Data Protection Act 1998. See www.opsi.gov.uk/ACTS/acts1998/19980029.htm or www.dh.gov.uk/PolicyAndGuidance/OrganisationPolicy/RecordsManagement/Data ProtectionAct1998 concerning its application to the NHS.

Department of Health. *Reference Guide to Consent for Examination or Treatment*. London: DoH; 2002.

Department of Health and Social Security. *Informed Consent*. DHSS Circular. HC. 1990; **90**(22).

Dyregrow A. *A Grief in Childhood: a handbook for adults*. London: Jessica Kingsley; 1991.

Ellershaw J, Wilkinson S. *Care of the Dying: A pathway to excellence*. Oxford: Oxford University Press; 2003.

Ellis PM, Tattersall MH. How should doctors communicate the diagnosis of cancer to patients? *Ann Med*. 1999; **31**(5): 336–41.

Evans J. Clinical negligence in NHS and the Law. *Wellard's NHS Handbook 1999/2000*. London: JHM Publishing; 1999.

Faulkner A. *When the News is Bad: a guide for health professionals*. Cheltenham: Stanley Thornes; 1998.

Fogarty LA, Curbow BA, Wingard JR *et al*. Can 40 seconds of compassion reduce patient anxiety? *J Clin Oncol*. 1999; **17**(1): 371–9.

Gillon R. Telling the truth and medical ethics. *BMJ*. 1985; **291**: 1556–7.

Girgis A, Sanson-Fisher RW. Breaking bad news 1: current best advice for clinicians. *Behav Med*. 1998; **24**(2): 53–9.

General Medical Council (GMC). *Consent: patients and doctors making decisions together*. London: General Medical Council; 2008. See link at www.gmc-uk.org or go to www.gmc-uk.org/guidance/ethical_guidance/consent_guidance/Consent_guidance.pdf

General Medical Council (GMC). *Maintaining Boundaries*. London: General Medical Council; 2006.

General Medical Council (GMC). *Withholding and Withdrawing Life Prolonging Treatments: good practice in decision making*. London: General Medical Council; 2002.

Health and Safety at Work Act 1974. See www.hse.gov.uk or www.pcs.org.uk, www.healthandsafety.co.uk or www.opsi.gov.uk or just Google search for the Act.

Heegaard M. *When Someone Very Special Dies: children can learn to cope with grief*. Minneapolis, MN: Woodland; 1991.

Heegaard M. *When Something Terrible Happens: children can learn to cope with grief*. Minneapolis, MN: Woodland; 1991.

Hippocrates. Decorum, XVI. In: Jones WH. *Hippocrates with an English translation. Vol II*. London: William Heinemann; 1923.

Human Rights Act 1998, Article 2 'Right to Life', Article 3 'Right to be Free from Inhuman or Degrading Treatment', Article 8 'Right to Respect for Privacy & Family Life', Article 10 'Freedom of Expression', Article 14 'Freedom from Discriminatory Practices'.

Job N. *Childhood Bereavement: developing the curriculum and pastoral support*. London: National Children's Bureau; 2004.

Jurkovich GJ, Pierce B, Pananen L *et al*. Giving bad news: the family perspective. *J Trauma*. 2000; **48**(5): 865–70.

Levine M, Pyke J. *Levine on Coroners' Courts*. London: Sweet & Maxwell; 1998.

McDermott MB. Obtaining consent for autopsy. *BMJ*. 2003; **327**: 804–6.

McLauchlan CA. Handling distressed relatives and breaking bad news. *BMJ*. 1990; **301**(6761): 1145–9.

Medical Defence Union publications: *Can I see the Records, Confidentiality, Consent to Treatment, The MDU Guide to the Complaints Procedure, Problems in General Practice – delay in diagnosis, Clinical Negligence, Inquests – a practical medico-legal guide, GP Registrars – a practical medico-legal guide*. London: MDU.

Ministry of Justice. *Cremation Regulations 2008: guidance for doctors*. Ministry of Justice; 2008.

Mitchell JL. Cross-cultural issues in the disclosure of cancer. *Cancer Pract*. 1998; **6**(3): 153–60.

Neuberger J. *Caring for Dying People of Different Faiths*. 2nd ed. London: Mosby; 1991.

NHS. *NHS Guidelines: patients who die in hospital.* HSG(92). London: Department of Health; 1992.

NHS. *Guidance on the Role and Effective Use of Chaperones in Primary and Community Care Settings: model chaperone framework.* London: NHS Clinical Governance Support Team, Department of Health; 2005.

NHS Litigation Authority website at www.nhsla.com

NHSE. *A Guide to Consent for Examination.* London: NHS Executive; 1990.

NPSA. *Being Open – communicating patient safety incidents with patients, their families and carers.* Available online at: www.nrls.npsa.nhs.uk/resources/?entryid45=65077

NPSA. *Being Open – supporting information.* Available online at: www.nrls.npsa.nhs.uk/resources/?entryid45=65077

NPSA. *Being Open – framework.* Available online at: www.nrls.npsa.nhs.uk/resources/?entryid45=65077

O'Grady G. Death of the teaching autopsy. *BMJ.* 2003; **327**: 802–3.

Parker PA, Baile WF, de Moor C *et al.* Breaking bad news about cancer: patients' preferences for communication. *J Clin Oncol.* 2001; **19**(7): 2049–56.

Ptacek JT, Eberhardt TL. Breaking bad news: a review of the literature. *JAMA.* 1996; **276**(6): 496–502.

Quill TE, Arnold RM, Platt F. 'I wish things were different': expressing wishes in response to loss, futility, and unrealistic hopes. *Ann Intern Med.* 2001; **135**(7): 551–5.

RCGP, BMA. *Preparing for Pandemic Influenza.* London: Royal College of General Practitioners and British Medical Association; December 2008 (published January 2009).

Report of the Joint Working Party of the Royal College of Pathologists, the Royal College of Physicians of London and the Royal College of Surgeons of England. *The Autopsy and Audit.* RCPath, RCP and RCS; 1991. Available online at Resuscitation Council website www.resus.org.uk

The Royal Marsden Hospital Manual of Clinical Nursing Procedures. 7th ed. London: Wiley Blackwell; 2008.

Underwood J. Commentary: resuscitating the teaching autopsy. *BMJ.* 2003; **327**: 803–4.

VandeKieft GK. Breaking bad news. *Am Fam Physician.* 2001; **64**(12): 1975–8.

Walsh RA, Girgis A, Sanson-Fisher RW. Breaking bad news 2: what evidence is available to guide clinicians? *Behav Med.* 1998; **24**(2): 61–72.

Research

The aim of this chapter is to provide an outline of current views and attitudes to research in the NHS generally and in training posts and give you an outline of ways that you could undertake research if you feel inclined to do so. It is not a step-by-step guide on how to undertake research, although hopefully some of the sources given in the related reading list at the end of the chapter might do so.

Research at national level

The UK Government spends over £1.5 billion on medical research every year and innovation in UK health research has risen in prominence in the last few years through two major government-commissioned reports. The first (Cooksey 2006), a review to build agreement on the best arrangements for the new single fund for health research, concluded that there was slow translation of research findings into health and economic benefit. This led to the formation of the Office for the Strategic Coordination of Health Research (OSCHR), set up to facilitate efficient translation of research into health through better strategic co-ordination of health research and more coherent funding arrangements, and in 2007 the government announced that funding for health research would rise to £1.7 billion per annum by 2010–11.

The main strategic aims of OSCHR are to:

o encourage alignment of the Medical Research Council (MRC), National Institute for Health Research (NIHR) and other government-funded health research strategies with a single integrated strategy for all health research
o promote effective cross-working between government agencies and retain clarity for the research community
o eliminate unnecessary duplication
o enhance capacity for translational and public health research
o enhance the partnership with industry and charity.

The report can be downloaded from www.hm-treasury.gov.uk/d/pbr06_cooksey_final_report_636.pdf.

The second report, *The Next Stage Review: high quality care for all* (Darzi 2008) suggested a change in the fundamental principle of how the health service is organised, with quality central to the delivery of patient care. Within this report there was a renewed focus on innovation through the setting up of the Health Innovation Council in 2009, designed to act as an overarching guardian for innovation from discovery through to adoption, holding the DoH and the NHS to account for helping to overcome barriers and taking up innovation. The Council's work is closely linked to the work of primary care trusts and practice-based commissioning. There are also other incentives to improve the translation of research and innovation into new treatments and techniques that would benefit patients. The report can be downloaded from www.dh.gov.uk/en/Managingyourorganisation/Commissioning/Worldclasscommissioning/DH_085747.

The DoH established the National Institute for Health Research (NIHR) in 2006 to provide the framework for publicly funded health research in England following publication of *Best Research for Best Health: a new national health research strategy* (DoH 2006). Its role is to manage and administer research programmes funded by the NIHR and the Department of Health that investigate a range of healthcare matters and assist in how research-based knowledge is applied across all healthcare sectors. Its principal function is to operate an online application facility and peer-review process to commission health research, underpinned by patient and public involvement. You can access the NIHR website at www.nihr-ccf.org.uk/site/default.cfm.

The National Institute for Health Research also introduced a Comprehensive Clinical Research Network (CCRN) in 2007 as a way to provide infrastructure for clinical trials in all areas of disease and clinical need within the NHS.

The CCRN was created as part of the government's research and development strategy as set out in *Best Research for Best Health: a new national health research strategy* (last modified in 2009) to provide a world-class infrastructure for clinical trials in all areas of disease and clinical need within the NHS. The document can be viewed at www.dh.gov.uk/en/Researchanddevelopment/Researchanddevelopmentstrategy/DH_4127109.

The aims of CCRN are to:

○ ensure that patients and healthcare professionals from all parts of the country and from all areas of healthcare can take part in and benefit from clinical research
○ improve the quality, speed and co-ordination of clinical research by removing the barriers to research within the NHS
○ streamline and performance manage NHS support for clinical studies to ensure that the costs of research are met in a timely and efficient manner
○ unify and streamline administrative procedures associated with regulation, governance, reporting and approvals
○ strengthen research collaboration with industry and ensure that the NHS can meet the health research needs of industry
○ further integrate health research and patient care.

Research at a personal level

Reliable, research-based information is fundamental to the successful implementation of clinical governance. This section provides only some general guidelines and insight into how to carry out research. It is not a tutorial on how to carry out research. Some suggestions for further reading may be found at the end of the chapter.

Engagement in the research fosters characteristics such as logical thought, critical analysis and self-reliance. These are of substantial benefit in clinical practice. Clinical practice can benefit greatly from research carried out by doctors with training in the methods and ethics of medical research. Most doctors who have undertaken periods of research would probably agree that they are better doctors for the experience. Research insight enables the interpretation and evaluation of research undertaken by others. It could be argued that all professional practice should be research-based and research-validated, providing not only patients with quality care and attention but also ensuring that those commissioning healthcare are getting value in the provision of the services. Training from research experience helps doctors to ask clinically relevant questions as well as directing the results of such experience towards better care of patients.

The problem now, however, is that whereas in the past knowledge of research and its methods were considered part of a broader educational experience for doctors in training, the move to quicker promotion from trainee to service provider has meant perhaps a loss of a valuable opportunity to be able to understand and appreciate and more so critically evaluate the relevance and value of experimental evidence presented to doctors. However, while the Gold Guide does still acknowledge the value of knowledge of research for trainees, this ideal and culture does not seem in practice to be very evident now and trainees undertaking higher degrees often experience criticism for having 'wasted their time'.

The Gold Guide on Research

The Guide to Postgraduate Specialty Training in the UK (2007), known as the Gold Guide, can be downloaded at www.jrcptb.org.uk/SiteCollectionDocuments/Gold%20 Guide.pdf. It devotes a number of pages in section 6 to the subject of academic training, research and higher degrees.

It states 'that all of the specialty training curricula require trainees to understand the value and purpose of medical research and to develop the skills required to critically assess research evidence'. Further, it states that some trainees will wish to consider or develop a career in academic medicine and may wish to explore this by undertaking a period of academic training (in either research or education) during their clinical training. The guide provides web links to important advice on pursuing an academic clinical career: either Academic Medicine at www.academicmedicine.ac.uk or NCCRCD – NIHR Trainees Coordinating Centre (part of the NHSNIHR) at www.nihrtcc.nhs. uk/?school_id=26.

Two main routes are suggested, either for opportunities to enter PMETB-approved integrated combined academic and clinical programmes, or to take time out of their deanery specialty training programme to undertake research or an appropriate higher degree (Out of Programme for Research – OOPR) with the agreement of the Postgraduate Dean. Trainees continue to hold their National Training Numbers (NTN) during this time out of their clinical programme.

A trainee can request deferral for up to three years before starting a run-through specialty training programme if they have been accepted to a higher degree programme (e.g. PhD, MD, MSc) at the time of being offered their clinical placement or if they are already undertaking research for a registered degree when their clinical placement is due to start. It also states that because of the short duration of training in general practice, deferral in this specialty is unlikely to be agreed.

Each of the four countries has developed or is in the process of developing their own arrangements for these integrated academic and clinical posts. So you would need to go to the appropriate website for further information.

When to research

With sufficient time, research can be performed readily. Most doctors research as part of an additional or higher degree; for example, an intercalated BSc, MSc, MD, MS/MCh, MPhil or PhD. The timeframe of these courses varies considerably and admission to such courses relates to clinical post, experience and interests. Particular attention must also be paid to funding and access to clinical posts upon completion of research.

Undertaking research

You are likely to be influenced by your planned area of specialisation, areas of special interest to you or questions already under study in the department in which you work. Interest and perceived importance of the topic are necessary in order to maintain motivation. You also need to ask yourself whether you can be unbiased in the chosen topic. There is little point in starting unless you are sure you can complete the project within the available time.

Research is usually divided into 'pure' and 'applied'. Pure research has as its first objective the advancement of knowledge and the understanding of the relations between variables. The researcher may not have any practical intention for the research, only the development of understanding. Because this type of research does not offer any apparent useable outcomes it can be difficult to raise funding. Applied research, on the other hand, is undertaken to solve specific, practical questions. Its purpose is to seek solutions, although it too can and often does raise further questions. Thus, the division between the two is seldom clear-cut. The difference between basic and applied research may be said to lie in the time span between research and reasonably foreseeable practical applications.

Research methods

The essential purpose of research is to produce some new knowledge. In medicine, this is likely to involve either exploratory or empirical research.

Exploratory research is conducted because a problem has not been clearly defined. It helps to determine the best research design, data collection method and selection of subjects. Exploratory research often relies on secondary research such as reviewing available literature and/or data, or qualitative approaches such as informal discussions with patients, clinical specialists, managers or other service users. Sometimes more formal methods such as in-depth interviews, focus groups, projective methods, case studies or pilot studies are employed. The result of exploratory research is not necessarily used for decision making, but they can provide significant insight into a situation.

Empirical research attempts to describe accurately the interaction between the researcher's data-collection 'tool' (which may be as simple as the human eye) and the entity being observed. The researcher is expected to calibrate their instrument by applying it to known standard objects and documenting the results before applying it to unknown objects.

In practice, the accumulation of evidence for or against any particular theory involves planned research design. Design is sometimes determined as much by the researcher's experience and preference as it is by the nature of the topic being researched. Differences can arise between those who adopt a quantitative, or positivist, model of testing theory and those who prefer to rely on qualitative methods which are more focused on generating theories and accounts. Positivists treat the social world as something that is external to the social scientist and waiting to be researched. They traditionally seek to minimise intervention in order to produce valid and reliable statistics. Qualitative researchers, on the other hand, believe that the social world is constructed by social agency and therefore any intervention by a researcher will affect social reality. They traditionally treat intervention as something that is necessary, often arguing that participation in the situation being researched can lead to a better understanding of the social dimension.

Research process

Generally, medical research is likely to follow an established structural process. Though the order of the stages may vary depending on the subject matter and researcher, the following steps are usually part of most formal research, both pure and applied.

- **Formulation of the topic:** this may be determined by organisational need or could arise out of the researcher's experience.
- **Setting up the hypothesis:** a hypothesis usually refers to a provisional idea whose merit needs evaluation. A hypothesis requires more work by the researcher in order to either confirm or disprove it. In due course, a confirmed hypothesis may become part of a theory or grow to become a theory itself.
- **An operational definition:** a description of something that determines its presence and quantity. It is an exact description of how to derive a value for a characteristic being measured. It includes a precise definition of the characteristic and how, specifically, data collectors are to measure the characteristic. The operational definition is used to remove ambiguity and ensure all data collectors have the same understanding and can independently measure or test for them at will.
- **Collecting data:** data is the plural of datum. A datum is a statement accepted at face value – a 'given'. A large class of practically important statements are measurements or observations of a variable. They are usually collected as numbers, words or images.

○ **Analysis of data:** this stage is determined by the topic, the nature of the hypothesis, the approach taken to data collection and the preferences of the researcher. Medical research outcomes are most often based on statistical analysis of data. Such analysis will be challenged if the researcher is unable to demonstrate that systematic bias was avoided in the research process, that the assessment was 'blind' (that the researcher could not have been influenced by any kind of performance bias) and that basic statistical procedures were followed (choice of sample size, duration and completeness of follow-up).

○ **Conclusion, revising of hypothesis:** a common misunderstanding is that a hypothesis can be proven. Instead, it may only be disproven. The hypothesis may survive several rounds of scientific testing and be widely thought of as true, but this is not the same as it having been proven. It would be better to say that it has yet to be disproved.

Research guidance

There is an Academic Medicine Group of the medical royal colleges for doctors in training who wish to undertake research as an integral part of a career in academic medicine. They have written *Guidelines for Clinicians Entering Research* (1997), published by the Royal College of Physicians of London. This 16-page booklet will provide you with answers to many basic questions, such as where to go for your research, whether some projects are more suitable than others, deciding on which degree is more suitable, funding, where to get advice, what happens after your research such as career re-entry and implications for new training arrangements for those in academic and research medicine. An appendix provides some useful contact addresses such as medical organisations and regional postgraduate deans, from whom further advice may be obtained. (Be aware, though, that is 12 years since it was published.)

The Walport Report 2005

This is so called because it was chaired by Dr Mark Walport, Director of The Wellcome Trust and published by a sub-committee of the UK Clinical Research Collaboration (UKCRC) and the NHS Modernising Medical Careers, and entitled *Medically- and Dentally-Qualified Academic Staff: recommendations for training the researchers and educators of the future.* The report made recommendations for initiatives to integrate the development of academic skills with each of the key stages of a clinician's career. It would be worth reading if you are seriously interested in research and an academic career in research.

Practical aspects of researching

This section is not a primer on undertaking research but guidance notes for those who are interested perhaps in publishing a paper and a pointer in the right direction for further action together with brief notes on a few key requirements. Specific provision is being made for those who wish to follow an academic career in medicine as

MMC includes an initiative to enhance academic training funding. This has been given to establish academic training programmes across all specialties. Trainees can enter these academic programmes from foundation into three-year Academic Clinical Fellowships (ACF). During this time they will be supported to acquire not only the clinical competences relevant to their specialty but also have protected research time to develop sufficient research expertise. They will then be in a position to apply for externally funded research grants. It is anticipated that trainees will then spend three years in funded research to gain a higher degree before returning to an Academic Clinical Lectureship (ACL) post to complete their training. This was hailed as good news for academic trainees that would hopefully reverse the decline in numbers of academic doctors that has been occurring in recent years.

You can read more about this in the Report of the Academic Careers Sub-Committee of Modernising Medical Careers and the UK Clinical Research Collaboration, *Medically- and Dentally-Qualified Academic Staff*, available online at www.nccrcd.nhs. uk/intetacatrain/index_html/copy_of_Medically_and_Dentally-qualified_Academic_ Staff_Report.pdf.

Others are expected to develop an understanding of research methodology and may wish to undertake some limited research if given an opportunity. Research can be enjoyable, but it is time-consuming, it can be expensive and is increasingly difficult unless you are pursuing an academic career path. In some ways it is like detective work, starting with a problem, going through a process of investigation, building up evidence and moving towards conclusions. The sense of achievement in new discovery can be tremendous, but beyond this personal satisfaction it could be argued that all professional practice should be research-based and research validated, and all professional doctors have a responsibility to contribute to the process.

GMC and principles governing research practice

- ○ When conducting research involving patients, the benefits of the research are not always certain. You must be sure that the research is not contrary to their interests. In particular you must ensure that, in therapeutic research, the risks do not outweigh the potential benefits. The development of treatments and furthering of knowledge should never take precedence over the patients' best interests. In non-therapeutic research, you must keep the risks to participants as low as possible. In addition, the potential benefits from the development of treatments and furthering of knowledge must far outweigh any such risks. Even research based on records that do not involve patients or volunteers directly requires following the basic ethical principles set out in their guidance. You should, whether the research is within the NHS, a university, the pharmaceutical industry, or elsewhere
- ○ ensure you have ethical approval from a properly constituted and relevant research ethics committee
- ○ conduct research in an ethical manner and in accordance with best practices
- ○ ensure that patients or volunteers understand that they are being asked to participate in research and that results can be unpredictable

o obtain and record the participants' consent; except in exceptional circumstances where specific approval not to obtain consent must have been given by the research ethics committee
o respect participants' right to confidentiality
o with participants' consent, keep GPs and other clinicians responsible for participants' care informed
o provide GPs with any information necessary for their care
o complete, or ensure others complete, research projects involving patients or volunteers
o record and report results accurately
o be prepared to explain and justify your actions and decisions
o be satisfied that you have appropriate authority to access identifiable data.

GMC and confidentiality

The GMC have sent all doctors a booklet entitled *Confidentiality* (GMC 2009) that contains advice on this issue in relation to research that ought to be read before undertaking clinical research, not only with patients but with medical records.

Informed consent is the obvious problem when anonymised data is not practical. And what can you do when patients cannot be traced? In England and Wales the National Information Governance Board (NIGB) (www.nigb.nhs.uk) may be able to assist, although not in Scotland and Northern Ireland.

Another possibility is the 'honest broker' approach as recommended by the Care Record Development Board's secondary uses working group in 2007. There is already such a situation in Scotland with the Information Services Division of the Common Services Agency in NHS Scotland (www.nhsnss.org/pages/divisions/information_ services_division.php) able to consider and authorise disclosures for purposes such as research.

Keeping up with the literature

With so many published journals how do you keep up to date with the literature, especially if you are involved in writing or research? Well, for a start keeping up to date goes beyond just reading publications and attending meetings. It is just as important to be able to recall articles quickly, to cite references accurately and to quote from them correctly. To make this easier, you need to do three things:
o acquire the information
o note the important information
o store references so they can be easily retrieved.

Acquiring information

Your choice of reading depends of course on your research and general interests. It will cover journals, books, conference and other reports, especially review articles and journals that review papers published within a specialty each month. Do not forget that scanning the index of journals will give you a good idea of published material. If you need to do a detailed study or review of a subject you should search computerised bibliographic databases such as Medline, about which your librarian can give you advice. See also literature reviews. From such databases you will obtain citations of all your references, and, in many cases, abstracts. How much time you spend reading new material each week depends on the time you have and the amount of reading you need to do.

Noting important information

This used to be done manually with record cards, although people would now use a computer database. You will need to record:
o title of the paper
o authors
o full title of the journal or book
o volume number, page numbers and year of publication
o description of the paper and work (case report or general report, leading article, editorial, review or letter; results of controlled trial, original study)
o institution where the work was carried out
o key words
o an abstract
o location of material (e.g. your own collection, in the library, etc.).

Is the information relevant and valid?

Ask yourself the following questions when evaluating the research of others.
o Is it relevant for your project?
o Have rigorous, systematic and objective methods been used? The research should offer the highest quality evidence. For example, were participants in the study randomly selected or randomly assigned to experimental versus control/comparison? Was there a control group?
o Are there other possible explanations for the results that are reported in the research study or how they were interpreted by the authors?
o Is there sufficient detail for replication? The research should be described in enough detail so that other researchers can replicate the study.
o Has it been submitted to independent, expert review? There should be evidence that the research was reviewed by research and content experts, other than the researchers. A typical form of expert review would be publication in a refereed journal.

Storing information for retrieval

This is the most difficult of the three tasks but the most important. Your ability to recall the important message from the paper without necessarily reading it all over again will depend on how you file the information. A database is only an electronic filing cabinet, an organised collection of data on a given subject. The database will be composed of a single data file or several files – a file being a collection of records on a theme. All the records on a given subject make up a file, and all the files together form the database.

The record is divided into 'data fields', each holding information on one aspect of the reference, such as the names of the authors, as above. One advantage of the computer database is the ability to search for records on multiple variables, to create index files and to use the system in conjunction with word processing programs. You can either create your own system using the database supplied with your computer software or purchase a separate, more sophisticated package specially designed to handle bibliographic data. These are more expensive but some can communicate with bibliographic databases such as Medline and therefore provide means of obtaining a large number of references from the computer terminal installed in the department or even at home.

Getting published

Although the practical aspects of writing for publication has in the past been dealt with in Chapter 3 (that in earlier editions used to be 'Effective written communication') it has been suggested that readers would prefer all information related to research itself to appear in a separate chapter.

Publication in academic media is based on peer review before it is made available for a wider audience. Medical specialties generally have their own journals and other outlets for publication. Some journals are interdisciplinary, and publish work from several distinct fields or subfields. The kinds of publications that are accepted as contributions of knowledge or research vary greatly between fields.

Higher, research-based qualifications and publications can be of great value when applying for jobs, particularly in some oversubscribed specialties. Not only do they represent an interest in improved patient care and scientific understanding, but also a desire to improve personal development. If an academic career beckons, research interests and publications in reputable refereed journals are an essential prerequisite.

Key stages in the writing process are:
o developing your idea
o background reading and literature search
o conducting the research
o analysing the results
o writing.

Literature searches

One way to review the literature is to work laboriously backwards through the journals; either scanning the contents lists for suitable papers or reading some of the review journals. The modern, more efficient and easier way is to visit The National Library of Medicine (NLM) and enter the topic in the 'search' box at www.nlm.nih.gov/tsd/serials/lji.html.

The US NLM Pub Med search service at www.ncbi.nlm.nih.gov offers free and easy access to the old *Index Medicus* citations, or you can join any one of a variety of 'for a fee' commercial products that also provide this information. The Internet is now the almost universal way of searching the literature. If you are serious about doing online searches and downloading data from your computer at home you will need broadband.

The Doctors.net website is another place to start, although your own medical school, the postgraduate medical centre, local medical school or university will also be easy sources to use. In addition, many universities and medical royal colleges have facilities, although in these latter cases you may need to register. Below are a few sites to help you commence your search.

Doctors.net alone will access the following.

- Medline, an invaluable resource for health science professionals. Many of the references in this book were checked on this source.
- Dove Medical Press, with access to 76 medical journals.
- Encyclopaedia Britannica, the oldest and largest general reference in the English language, with more than 70,000 articles and free abstracts for members.
- *PLoS Medicine*, an open-access, peer-reviewed journal published monthly by the Public Library of Science. PLoS Medicine publishes the most significant advances in all medical disciplines, including epidemiology and public health.
- *Merck Manual of Diagnosis and Therapy*, full text of the 17th (Centennial) edition.
- OMNI, a free UK-based gateway to resources in medicine, biomedicine, allied health and related topics.
- *BMJ*, published material for doctors and medical students. Subscriptions are required for the full text of some articles. Some of the older articles are freely available after a period of time or a particular article may have been made available in the public interest.
- *The Lancet*, a journal of review, news and opinion fully accessible through free registration.
- *JAMA*, a subscription is required for full text articles.
- *NEJM*, the oldest continuously published medical journal in the world. A subscription is required for full text articles.

There are online textbooks at Doctors.net:
- *Oxford Textbook of Rheumatology*
- *Oxford Textbook of Clinical Nephrology*
- *Oxford Textbook of Medicine*
- *Oxford Textbook of Psychiatry*
- *Oxford Textbook of Geriatric Medicine*.

There is also a patient information section with examples of leaflets explaining conditions and treatment to patients. This extensive library enables you to print leaflets off for you to give to your patients.

Most of the medical royal colleges have libraries with Internet search facilities but vary in the amount of text available, other than abstracts. Many universities and medical schools have similar facilities but most require you to register with them and use passwords.

From the above sources you will obtain citations, in many cases abstracts, and in a few cases copies of articles of your references. Your first attempts can often be frustrating and if you can obtain the help of a qualified librarian or an experienced colleague then do so. You first need to precisely define your search subject. Are there synonyms? Alternative spellings? (particularly if searching American sources) You also need to decide how far back you want the search to go. The further back you search, the more you will find, the less likely you are to get copies online and so the more time-consuming it becomes. Good research needs a framework or a set of stages, not necessarily chronological, which should be addressed systematically whatever the scale of the project. Choosing the topic and formulating the problem that is feasible within the timescale is just the beginning.

Information technology in research

The increasing use of electronic media in medicine produces problems with confidentiality and data protection with regard to letters, results systems, clinic schedules, digital photography, radiology pictures, virtual consultations via the web, and email.

There are some basic rules consistent with current advice that applies to all these situations.

o Computers must be physically secure and away from public access.
o Monitors must be placed so their screens face away from public view.
o All data must be password protected.
o Staff with access must be aware of their duty of confidentiality.
o Data can only be transmitted via the Internet with suitable encryption.
o Printouts should be treated as confidential and re-filed in a patient's notes or destroyed after use.

This means that data on a laptop is secure only if it is kept in a locked office, it does not leave the building and it has a password lock. You cannot take your laptop home with identifiable patient data on it. Information on computers will not be removed completely from the hard disc, even when deleted. Accidental deletions are a recurrent topic on the Doctors.net computing forum, and software is readily downloadable to restore lost files. There are programmes that can make the hard drive impossible to read, but destroying the hard drive is the only really sure method.

Junior doctors and data protection

Junior doctors who make personal records of patient data, such as for training logbook purposes, should be aware of the provisions of the Data Protection Act. If patient data is recorded on, for example, personal computers, and that data can identify a patient, the data must be held subject to the provisions of the Data Protection Act. This would require the doctor to be registered for this purpose. Furthermore, the transfer of such data between trusts is a breach of the Data Protection Act.

The BMA therefore advises junior doctors not to record the data with the patient's name, though data that can be matched to a patient only through use of a hospital record system or separate second data set is lawful on an unregistered computer. For example, a hospital number can only identify a patient if cross-referred with the hospital records system. It is probably wise to consult your medical royal college if you feel you are at risk of being in breach of the Act. Manual records have also been within the scope of the Data Protection Act since March 2000.

Developing IT skills

Most doctors, particularly those still in training, are now conversant with IT skills. For most trainees computer literacy is an essential part of their work, career development and record keeping. Developing the necessary skills for older doctors to make best personal use of IT requires more of an investment in time than in equipment and the earlier the investment is made the greater the potential benefit. You will have a real need to use IT for a research project. This is likely to provide the necessary motivation to complete the learning and integrate it into practice. Essential components are a period of structured training, access to technology and a clear goal to attain relevant IT skills as part of the project. A combination of books, perhaps local courses and direct supervision allow you to focus on skills that are most useful to your project. Progression from simpler tasks (e.g. email, word processing and slide presentations) towards the more complex (e.g. spreadsheets, databases and project management) provides positive feedback and avoids frustration. Some trusts encourage staff to study for and obtain the European Computer Driving License (ECDL). This is a distance-learning course designed to provide participants with competence in all of the main packages available on work-based computers.

Starting the written stages
Aims, objectives or hypotheses

Set out what you want to achieve and how. This will influence your choice of methodological approach and design of the study. The purpose of the research can be set out as a statement of aims or as a research hypothesis, or both. In health research the range of possible methodologies is vast, stretching from classical quantitative or scientific methods through a variety of structured and semi-structured designs and surveys to qualitative approaches. You also need to identify resource implications and may need to seek approval from your local ethics committee.

Pilot study for data collection

Having planned the study, including your forms for data recording, questionnaires, attitude scales, equipment needed to detect flaws in design, etc., a pilot study is essential. When happy with this you can then proceed to full data collection.

Preparation for writing

Having carried out all the work you then need to prepare the data for analysis and present the findings in a structured way. It might be helpful to reread the section on writing reports (*see* Chapter 5). It is also helpful to evaluate and reflect on how the research was carried out and whether some parts could have been done differently or better. The research process can be thought of as a cycle, where having worked through all stages you may well find yourself back at the beginning, rethinking the topic and formulation of the study. Each stage is interconnected with every other stage. For example, inadequate funding may mean revision of the scope of the project. To obtain an overview of the process it is helpful to consider each stage independently.

For more detailed and practical guidance on writing and constructing your paper, dissertation or thesis, you may find it helpful to read the section on 'Getting published' and 'Writing journal articles' in Chapter 5.

Related reading

Academic Medicine Group. *Guidelines for Clinicians Entering Research*. London: Royal College of Physicians of London; 1997.

Albert T. Effective writing. In: A White (ed.) *Textbook of Management for Doctors*. London: Churchill Livingstone; 1996. (Useful tips on style and grammar.)

Albert T. *A–Z of Medical Writing*. London: BMJ Books; 2000.

Albert T. *Write Effectively: a quick course for busy health workers*. Oxford: Radcliffe Publishing; 2008.

Albert T. *Winning the Publications Game*. 3rd ed. Oxford: Radcliffe Publishing; 2009.

Buzan T. *The Ultimate Book of Mind Maps*. London: Thorsons; 2005.

Buzan T. *Use Your Head: innovative learning and thinking techniques to fulfil your potential*. London: BBC Active; 2006.

Buzan T, Buzan B. *The Mind Map Book*. New York: Penguin; 1996.

Cooksey D. *A Review of UK Health Research Funding*. London: HMSO; 2006. Can be downloaded at www.hm-treasury.gov.uk/d/pbr06_cooksey_final_report_636.pdf

Darzi A. *NHS Next Stage Review. High quality care for all: NHS Next Stage Review Final Report*. London: Department of Health; 2008. Can be downloaded at www.dh.gov.uk/en/Managingyourorganisation/Commissioning/Worldclasscommissioning/DH_085747

Department of Health. *Research and Development in the New NHS*. London: DoH, HMSO; 1994.

Department of Health. *Best Research for Best Health: a new national health research strategy*. London: DoH; 2006. This and a raft of associated publications can be downloaded at www.dh.gov.uk/en/Researchanddevelopment/Researchanddevelopmentstrategy/DH_4127109

GMC. *Confidentiality*. London: General Medical Council; 2009.

Gosall NK, Gosall G. *The Doctor's Guide to Critical Appraisal*. Knutsford: PasTest Ltd; 2006.

Greenhalgh T. How to read a paper: the Medline database. *BMJ*. 1997; **315**(7108): 596–9.

Greenhalgh T. *How to Read a Paper: the basics of evidence-based medicine*. 3rd ed. Oxford: Wiley-Blackwell and BMJ Books; 2006.

Murrell G, Huang C, Ellis H. *Research in Medicine*. 2nd ed. Cambridge: Cambridge University Press; 1999.

National Institute for Health Research. *Bureaucracy Busting: the research passport and streamlined HR arrangements*. London: DoH; 2009. Available online at www.nihr.ac.uk/files/pdfs/Implementation Plan 4.1d Bureaucracy Busting. Research Passport and streamlined HR arrangements.pdf

Paton A. *Write a Paper: how to do it 1*. 2nd ed. London: BMJ Books; 1985.

Phillips EM, Pugh DS. *How to Get a PhD: a handbook for students and their supervisors*. 4th ed. Maidenhead: Open University Press; 2005.

Report of the Academic Careers Sub-Committee of Modernising Medical Careers and the

UK Clinical Research Collaboration. *Medically- and Dentally-Qualified Academic Staff: recommendations for training the researchers and educators of the future.* London: UKCRC and MMC; 2005.

Royal College of Surgeons Policy Seminar. *Research in Surgery.* London: The Royal College of Surgeons of England; March 2009. Available online at www.rcseng.ac.uk/policy/ policy-seminars/research-in-surgery

Sackett DL, Rosenberg WMC, Gray JAM, Haynes RB. Evidence-based medicine: what it is and what it isn't. *BMJ.* 1996; **312**: 71–2.

The Walport Report. *Medically- and Dentally-qualified Academic Staff: recommendations for training the researchers and educators of the future.* Report of the Academic Careers Sub-committee of the UK Clinical Research Collaboration. London: UK Clinical Research Collaboration and Modernising Medical Careers; 2005. It can be downloaded from the *BMA* website if you are a member, or online at www.nihrtcc.nhs.uk/intetacatrain/index_ html/copy_of_Medically_and_Dentally-qualified_Academic_Staff_Report.pdf

Index